Suspicious Death Scene Investigation

Suspicious Death Scene Investigation

Edited by

PETER VANEZIS

MD, PhD, FRCPath, DMJ (Path)

Regius Professor of Forensic Medicine and Science,
The University of Glasgow, Glasgow, UK

ANTHONY BUSUTTIL

MD, FRCPath, DMJ (Path), FRCP Ed, FRCP Glas

Regius Professor of Forensic Medicine,
The University of Edinburgh, Edinburgh, UK

A member of the Hodder Headline Group
LONDON • SYDNEY • AUCKLAND
Co-published in the USA by Oxford University Press, Inc., New York

First published in Great Britain 1996 by
Arnold, a member of the Hodder Headline group,
338 Euston Road, London NW1 3BH

Co-published in the United States of America by
Oxford University Press, Inc.
198 Madison Avenue, New York, NY 10016
Oxford is a registered trademark of Oxford University Press

Whilst the advice and information in this book is believed to be true and
accurate at the date of going to press, neither the authors nor the publisher
can accept any legal responsibility or liability for any errors or omissions
that may be made. In particular (but without limiting the generality of the
preceding disclaimer) every effort has been made to check drug dosages;
however, it is still possible that errors have been missed. Furthermore,
dosage schedules are constantly being revised and new side-effects
recognized. For these reasons the reader is strongly urged to consult the
drug companies' printed instructions before administering any of the drugs
recommended in this book.

British Library Cataloguing in Publication Data
A catalogue record for this book is available from the British Library

Library of Congress Cataloging-in-Publication Data
A catalog record for this book is available from the Library of Congress

ISBN 0 340 55863 6 (hb)

Typeset in 10/11 Times by
Keyboard Services, Luton, Bedfordshire
Printed and bound in Great Britain by
St Edmundsbury Press, Bury St Edmunds, Suffolk

Contents

Contents

Contributors

Anthony Busuttil Regius Professor of Forensic Medicine, University of Edinburgh, Edinburgh, UK, and Chairman of the European Council for Legal Medicine

Zakaria Erzinçlioglu Visiting Scholar, Department of Zoology, University of Cambridge, Cambridge, UK

David Halliday Team Leader, Fire Investigation Unit, The Metropolitan Police Forensic Science Laboratory, London, UK

Pamela Hamer Trace Analysis Expert, The Metropolitan Police Forensic Science Laboratory, London, UK

Allan Parker Formerly Senior Photographer, Photographic Section, New Scotland Yard, London, UK

David Pryor Firearms Expert, The Metropolitan Police Forensic Science Laboratory, London, UK

Ray Ruddick Senior Forensic Photographer, Department of Forensic Medicine, The London Hospital Medical College, London, UK

David Sanderson Laboratory Liaison Officer, Detective Sergeant, Metropolitan Police, London, UK

Peter Vanezis Regius Professor of Forensic Medicine and Science, University of Glasgow, Glasgow, UK

Elizabeth Wilson Section Manager, Biology Division, The Metropolitan Police Forensic Science Laboratory, London, UK

Preface

A number of excellent texts on crime scene investigation are available but, to the best of our knowledge, none that concentrates solely on suspicious death scene investigation. When putting pen to paper our aim was not to attempt to replace the broadly based scene books but rather to supplement them, and, it is hoped, to add a new perspective, specifically from the standpoint of the forensic pathologist, which was inevitable, bearing in mind the pathological bias of both of us.

There are a number of contributors with whom we have worked on cases over the years, all experienced and expert in their particular field to whom we are extremely grateful and without whom the production of the text would not have been possible. One interesting aspect of putting together this text was that the interdisciplinary nature of the expertise required in scene work became readily apparent, thus it was not possible to confine some of the contributors to the section they were requested to write, because of the amount of overlap between us all. We have therefore exercised a degree of flexibility in transferring different contributors' material, where appropriate, to sections other than their own.

The text is divided into two broad sections. The first part deals with the different aspects of scene examination and the second part examines the scene in relation to different types of deaths. We have liberally cited cases because we believe strongly that this is the easiest way to put over an important point.

We also tried to avoid too much duplication of material covered in standard forensic pathology textbooks and so there is strict adherence to the procedure at the scene. We have thus refrained from any detailed description of other investigations that have to be carried out once the body is taken to the mortuary, except where such procedures assist in explaining the reasons for that specific aspect of scene investigation. We hope that the readers will find the book of practical value.

Our main aim has been to try to focus the reader's mind on the guiding principles of scene investigation and to appreciate fully the 'teamwork' approach that is essential for a successful outcome. As we are all aware, the type and scope of scenes and their assessment can vary enormously from case to case, and all investigators must be prepared to meet any challenge in his or her quest for truth and accuracy with a modicum of common sense and careful management. Only in this way may the interests of justice be properly and fully served.

P. Vanezis
A. Busuttil
March 1996

Acknowledgements

We would like to thank the following for permission to publish photographic material from cases: The Commissioner of the Metropolitan Police, and Chief Constables of Kent, Sussex, Hertfordshire, Bedfordshire, West Midlands and Lincolnshire. We also thank Dr Brian Pitkin, Natural History Museum, London, for allowing us to publish the line drawings of insects in Chapter 6. Line drawings have also been used in certain cases to replace photographic prints which were deemed by one particular Constabulary to be too sensitive for publication in their original form.

PART 1

Scene Examination

CHAPTER 1

General principles of scene examination

Introduction

One of the most crucial, if not *the* most crucial, aspect of the investigation of a suspicious death, is the comprehensive examination of the place of discovery of the body – the scene. Its assessment, together with the collection of all relevant samples and their examination, will facilitate the investigators' quest to establish accurately the circumstances surrounding the death in question.

When a body is discovered it is the task of the forensic investigators to determine firstly whether or not one is dealing with homicide. In the majority of cases, assessment of the type of death one is dealing with is reasonably straightforward. However, in a significant number of cases, the cause and manner of death may not be immediately obvious and, unless investigators adopt a low threshold of suspicion and treat all cases as potential homicides from the outset, serious errors can be made, which may be irredeemable. It is not difficult to imagine a situation where death is initially thought to be due to natural causes, and the scene and body barely considered in any detail, only to discover the bullet wound in the back at a later stage. All investigators are aware of such horror stories, where, to everyone's acute embarrassment, the first person to notice any injury to the body, especially on the back, has been the undertaker or the mortuary technician. The point is that one should not jump to conclusions in deaths where there is initially some suspicion, and injuries (or their full extent and nature) are not readily apparent or indeed where their appearance has been modified in some way. It is essential to wait until the autopsy has been completed, by which time in the vast majority of cases, the cause of death and the type of case one is dealing with will be clear. It is always better to assume the worst scenario and err on the side of caution. A slightly longer, albeit unnecessary investigation into a suicide that has been mistaken for a homicide is much more preferable to failure to initially investigate a homicide thoroughly (when the trail is hot) because it had been mistaken for a suicide.

Concept of the scene

It should be appreciated that the scene at which a body is found is quite often not where death occurred. It is not unusual for someone to have been killed at one locus and then deposited elsewhere. It becomes further complicated by the fact that an actual incident leading to death, e.g., stabbing, may have occurred in an entirely different location from where death occurred.

One should therefore appreciate that the scene of discovery of a body may be related to the actual incident leading to death and the place of death in a number of ways. Three common situations are illustrated in the following four examples.

CASE 1.1

A 35-year-old male prisoner who was serving a sentence for molesting a child, was struck repeatedly by a fellow inmate with a heavy metal pipe in his prison cell whilst lying asleep on his bed. The distribution and extent of blood spattering, caused by swinging the pipe at the deceased's head a number of times as well as a pool of blood, which was particularly heavy under the head region, clearly indicated that, after the

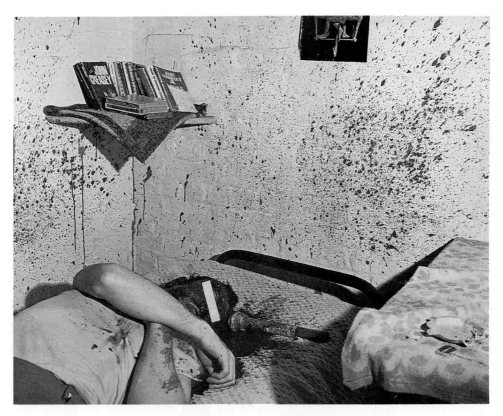

Figure 1.1   The deceased is shown *in situ* with the weapon, metal piping, by his head. The blood stain distribution on the adjacent walls of his prison cell clearly show that the fatal injuries and death occurred where he was found.

initial one or two blows, the deceased did not move from the position in which he was assaulted and subsequently found. In this case the scene of the assault leading to death was also the scene of death and where the body was discovered (Figure 1.1).

CASE 1.2
An 18-year-old male was stabbed outside the back of a public house. He then staggered down the road and leant on a car, which showed a few blood stains. He then continued a further 10 metres where he collapsed and died. It was initially thought that he had emerged from the house adjacent to where he was found (Figure 1.2(a) and 1.2(b)).

CASE 1.3
A 42-year-old female was found dead in a garage. She had been strangled by her husband in their house, which was about 100 metres away from where she was discovered. He then transported her to the garage during the night, using a wheelbarrow, and positioned her body and clothing so that it would be thought that she had been sexually assaulted then killed by another (Figure 1.3(a) and 1.3(b)).

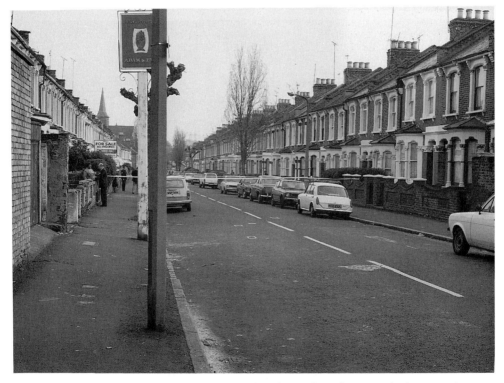

Figure 1.2(a) View from public house (bar) from where the victim had staggered after receiving the fatal stab wound. Note that the area where he was found is cordonned off with tape.

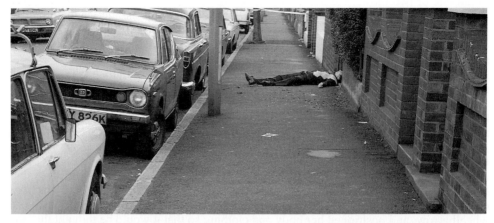

Figure 1.2(b) The deceased is shown lying across the pavement with his head by the front gate of the house from where it was originally thought that he had emerged.

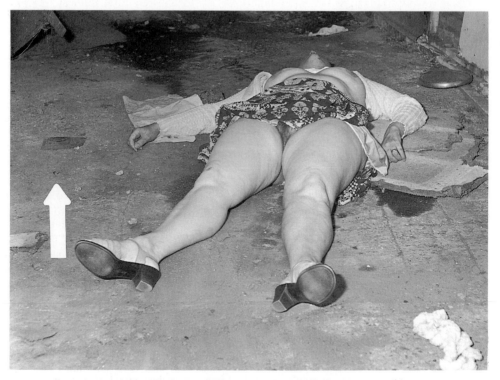

Figure 1.3(a) The body of a woman shown lying supine with her legs slightly parted. Her pants have been removed (shown in bottom right-hand corner), and a ring removed from her right hand and placed by her side (arrow). Her upper clothing has also been opened exposing her chest. There were no signs of a struggle on the body, which could be related to the scene of discovery.

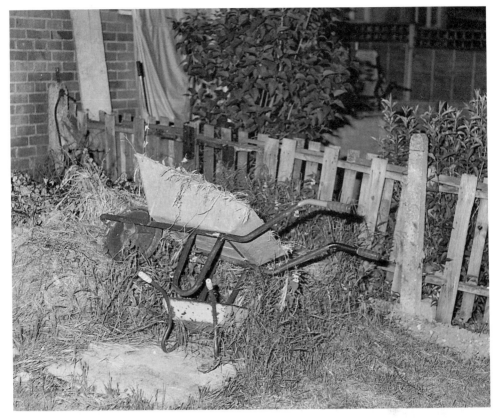

Figure 1.3(b) A discarded wheelbarrow used to transport the victim.

CASE 1.4

Six black plastic bin liners were discovered within dustbins outside a 'battered women's refuge' in East London. The bin liners contained six pieces of fresh human remains from one individual (Figure 1.4(a)). They comprised both lower legs, dismembered at the knees, both upper legs, dismembered at the hip joints, and both entire upper arms, dismembered at the shoulder joints. The liners containing them were neatly wrapped to seal the contents with a wide sealing tape. For five years their identification remained a mystery, despite extensive police enquiries and comprehensive forensic work, which identified them as being those of a female in her twenties, about 1.65 m (5' 6") in height, not pregnant, with traces of diazepam in her tissues. From her feet, she showed all the signs of having lead a fairly active life (these were examined in detail by a chiropodist) and she had multiple parallel old scars on both wrists indicating that she had at some stage attempted to commit suicide. The scene was unhelpful and indeed initially mislead the team into thinking that the premises were somehow relevant to her death and disposal.

The reality could not have been further from the truth. Five years later, it was discovered a young Irish man, recently settled in North West London and living in a flat in the same block as the deceased, met her (an Irish female in her early twenties) by chance, when she knocked on his door in error, looking for a friend. He struck up a

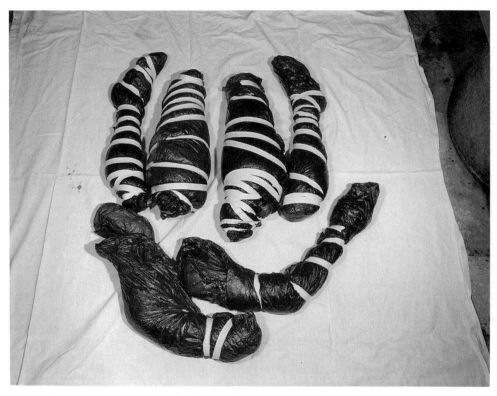

Figure 1.4(a) Dismembered limbs wrapped up in bin liners and secured with white adhesive tape. They were found stacked by some dustbins outside a terrace house used as a 'battered women's refuge'.

conversation with her then, after inviting her into his flat, tried to have sexual intercourse with her and then strangled her. He put her under his bed, went to sleep and woke up the next morning, incredulous at what he had done. He eventually removed her from under the bed and placed her near a radiator where she sustained some post-mortem burns as seen in Figure 1.4(b). He then dismembered her with a carving knife, placed her head and trunk into two bin liners in the dustbins outside the flat. These were taken away by refuse collectors, undetected, and disposed of in the normal way. The rest of the human remains, as there was no more room in the bins, he placed into two heavy-duty carrier bags, and took the London Underground train and crossed over to the East side of London to Mile End (the only other location in London that he knew). He then walked about half a mile and placed them, purely by chance, at the scene, where they were found soon after they were deposited.

In most investigators' experience, most commonly, the place where the person is killed is the same as that where the body is found.

The personal experience of one of us (PV) of 634 cases examined within the London area and the Home Counties, concerning the interrelationship between the scene of the fatal incident, death and discovery of the body, showed the following distribution:

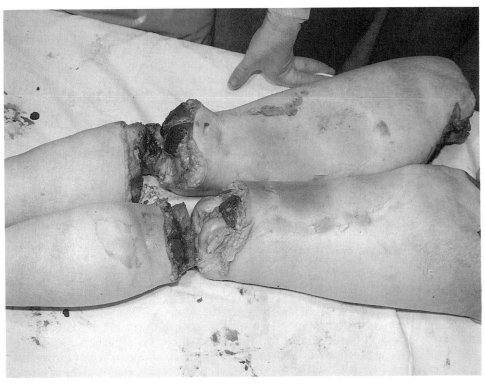

Figure 1.4(b) A view of the back of the legs. Note the post-mortem burning on the backs of both thighs and right lower leg near the back of the knee. These had been caused by placing the body close to a radiator with the legs straightened out before they were dismembered.

Scene of: Incident	Death	Discovery	n	%
Same	Same	Same	471	74
Different	Same	Same	123	20
Same	Same	Different	36	6

One of the greatest difficulties in an investigation, arises where there is an appreciable time lapse between the fatal incident and death. This is particularly pertinent, for example, in cases of head injury giving rise to a subdural haematoma, where death occurs after a lucid interval which may be days or weeks after the fatal injury. It may thus be extremely difficult or impossible to pinpoint the site and incident where the fatal injury occurred, particularly if the victim is prone to injury, for example, through alcohol abuse. The following is an example of such a case.

CASE 1.5
A 58-year-old male was struck on the face, propelling his head against the side of a car. He was apparently asymptomatic for about one week. He then began to develop photophobia and gradually worsening headache, and was found dead at his home about 24 hours after the onset of symptoms. Considerable difficulty was encountered in attempting to establish that the impact against the car was the fatal incident, given the time interval between that incident and death. The situation was further complicated by evidence that the deceased had stumbled over on other occasions before and after the alleged fatal incident.

There may also be an appreciable time lapse between death and disposal of a body. Zugibe and Costello (1993) reported on the investigation of a murder victim, one of a series of contract killings carried out by the notorious 'Iceman'. The deceased was found on a mountain road, wrapped with numerous layers of plastic garbage bags and rope. He had been killed by a gunshot wound to the head. It emerged from the investigations carried out that the body had been stored in a freezer for over two years before disposal.

Types of scene encountered

Scenes are so varied that one can only categorise them in very broad terms and, in some cases, in respect of the type of incident, e.g., a fire or an explosion. The type of scene encountered in practice will obviously depend to a great extent on the environment of one's catchment area, as well as various other geographical, sociological or human factors.

The examination of each type of scene, frequently requires a different type of approach, with the attendance of appropriate forensic expertise, depending very much on the type of location and/or type of incident. For example, the approach to a fire scene will be very different to the examination of a shallow grave in a back garden.

The importance of the 'scene team' and sound management practice

The investigation of a scene should be carried out by a team of professionals with well-defined functions and objectives, working in harmony. Indeed, the importance of the 'scene team' with a good team leader cannot be overstated. The examiner may only get one chance to collect the necessary evidence, which will be crucial to the successful outcome of the case. Awareness, therefore, of the importance of scene preservation and the correct procedures to follow throughout, is essential. The various police and forensic science establishments thoughout the United Kingdom publish their own thorough instructions for scene investigators. Relevant sections of the training manual produced by Lewington (1990) of the Metropolitan Police Forensic Science Laboratory as well as a basic list Scene of Crime Officers standard equipment may be found in the Appendices.

Management of the scene comprises the following essential components:

1. Searching for a body (if applicable).
2. Discovery of a body and preliminary assessment.
3. Appointing an investigating officer and forming a scene team, including relevant specialists.
4. Briefing before and/or after visit to the scene.
5. Health and safety considerations.
6. Scene assessment and collection of evidence.
7. Retrospective scene visit(s).

SEARCHING FOR A BODY

Where a search has been instigated to look for a body, substantial assistance both in manpower and equipment, occasionally of a highly specialised nature, may be required. This topic is discussed in more detail in Chapter 5.

DISCOVERY OF A BODY

When a body is discovered, the initial question that arises concerns the manner of death one is dealing with, particularly whether or not the death is suspicious, and, furthermore, who has the authority to arrive at such a conclusion.

The initial stage of discovery of a body is fraught with the potential for basic inappropriate actions, decisions and contamination. The person making the discovery, who in many cases is a member of the general public, may cause contamination, move an obviously dead body, attempt resuscitation where inappropriate and so on. This is occasionally also inadvertently done by the first police officer at the scene, who is often of low rank and has probably seen very few, if any, dead bodies *in situ* and thus is unaware of the requirements for scene preservation to the degree that an experienced detective officer would be. It is essential therefore that all officers are well trained to ensure that they do nothing more than preserve life, where necessary, then secure the scene and remain there to protect it from intruders, until the investigative team arrives.

ARRIVAL OF THE INVESTIGATING OFFICER AND PRELIMINARY ASSESSMENT

The investigating officer who is placed in charge of the enquiry (Collinson, 1970) will have full responsibility for the management of the scene, decide on the plan of action, set up an incident room and assemble the scene team, including any specialists who the officer may feel are relevant to the investigation, bearing in mind the particular circumstances of the case.

On arrival of the investigating officer at the scene, an assessment will be made as to whether or not any suspicion is attached to the death. In some cases this is a simple matter where advice may also be sought initially from the clinical forensic medical examiner (police surgeon), who is called to certify the fact of death. However, if there is doubt, then usually the investigating officer or a scene of crime officer will contact a pathologist to inform him or her of the circumstances. It should also be appreciated that other deaths that require special examination of the scene, may not involve a criminal offence but it may, nevertheless, be in the public interest for an investigation along such lines. In some such cases the definition of suspicion and whether or not a criminal offence has taken place, may be unclear; it is in such circumstances that there is the potential for mismanagement.

A successful scene investigation relies on teamwork and good scene management by the investigating officer in order that the various tasks are methodically attended to in a well-defined order of priority. In multiple deaths or potentially difficult and complicated cases, a briefing, which includes all the scene team, including the pathologist, should be held to discuss in detail the procedure to be adopted.

Obviously, the most urgent and prime consideration is to maintain life, if there is any chance that the victim may still be alive. Thus a doctor or paramedic may enter a scene to try to revive an injured person before any precautions are taken to prevent contamination of the body and its immediate environment. This action is beyond the control of the investigating officer but, once the person is pronounced dead, the scene should be secured and access restricted and monitored.

The senior investigator, when assessing a scene, must always, therefore, take into account:

1. *The location.* The body may be found in a dwelling or out of doors, buried in soil or recovered from water. Indeed, there are many possible types of locations. Furthermore, the investigating officer should appreciate that, as the investigation progresses, there may be the need for a number of locations to be examined, which relate to the same case. There are no hard and fast rules as to the number of loci that need to be examined in an enquiry. The more complicated a crime, the greater the likelihood that there will be an extensive list of locations that might need to be examined.

2. *Type of incident.* It is useful also to categorise scenes according to the type of incident because certain types of scene will require to be investigated by relevant teams or individuals with particular expertise and experience. The most obvious types of scenes where specialist investigators are necessary include those involving fires, explosions, firearms, industrial and tranportation accidents, and the discovery of skeletal remains.

3. *Number of deceased persons.* A particular scene at a particular time may be concerned with one body, although the possibility should always be borne in mind that, in the case of serial killings, multiple scenes may be related to one murderer or a single scene may also contain a number of deceased persons. A scene with multiple deaths may well be where death occurred, although, with clandestine mass graves, death may have occurred elsewhere and the bodies transported to the burial site.

4. *Health and safety.* This is discussed below.

5. *Urgency of the examination.* The location of the body may well necessitate urgent examination at the site and its removal to the mortuary. A body found by the seashore, for example, will need to be examined and moved before it is submerged by water as a result of tidal movement. A body may be in a busy thoroughfare, where it is therefore clearly undesirable to keep it there for any longer than necessary. Scene examination at night should be left to first light on the following morning if at all possible. The potential for misinterpreting the scene findings and indeed missing vital evidence is very real in poor lighting conditions.

6. *Climatic conditions.* The weather conditions prevailing at the scene may dictate the approach that needs to be adopted for investigation at the location. Adverse conditions may require the body to be moved to the mortuary as soon as

possible. If this cannot be done, then appropriate steps such as erecting a tent, should be taken to protect the body from the elements. In a particularly hot environment, for example, one should bear in mind that decomposition would be rapidly accelerated and the body should be removed at the earliest opportunity for autopsy or refrigerated.

7. *Available resources and expertise.* Clearly, there are marked differences in some areas as to the support that may be available. Nevertheless, cost effectiveness can be achieved by good organisation, careful preparation and good liaison between the team members.

8. *Security.* This is discussed below.

PROTECTING THE SCENE

Firstly, it must be decided what the boundaries of the scene are that need to be preserved. It is commonsense to start with as wide an area as possible and then contract it if necessary. This will depend on the circumstances, dictated by the location of the body and natural boundaries. The possibility of multiple scenes must also be borne in mind.

Securing an indoor scene such as a dwelling is usually a relatively straightforward matter; its limits are generally well defined. However, at the earliest stage, when knowledge of events may be incomplete or inaccurate, it is wise to secure as wide an area as possible, which can be contracted later. Cordonning off an area for examination is achieved in a number of ways, depending on the location, by placing clearly marked signs forbidding entry, ropes, barricades and additional manpower, particularly where there is the potential for intrusion into the scene by a large number of people, such as press, sightseers and so on.

Where the scene is out of doors, its protection may be more difficult. Apart from the use of physical barriers, it will, in many instances, be necessary to fence off a wide area in order to keep unauthorised persons well away. There may also need to be some aerial cover such as a tent over the body or even a marquee if one is dealing with multiple deaths, particularly to prevent unauthorised photography of the scene and of the deceased from long distances, high vantage points or from light aircraft.

Each member of the scene examination team has their own particular role, and must be aware of the each other's tasks and especially the need for preservation and collection of different types of evidence by the various specialist examiners. The pathologist, for example, must take account of the possibility of shoeprint evidence when entering a scene. It is essential that one scene examiner does not contaminate the scene for another. Furthermore, it is imperative that protective clothing be worn to protect the examiner from materials at the scene and also to protect the scene from the examiner. Each person should wear overalls, gloves and overshoes. It should be noted that overshoes will not prevent a scene examiner treading on shoeprints and scuffing away or transferring blood from one room to another. It is possible to use overshoes with a specific design printed on the sole so that it is clear that any shoeprints from these are fortuitous to the scene. All contaminated protective clothing must be disposed of properly after the scene examination. With modern, very sensitive analysis techniques, it is possible to contaminate a scene unintentionally. A scene examiner should not smoke and deposit ash at a scene. The examiner's clothing should not shed fibres at the scene. There may be traces of blood in the waste trap of a sink where the suspect has washed blood off, therefore the use of sinks and lavatories is forbidden.

It may be useful for the scene examiners to have a portable chair, particularly if they are going to spend some time observing blood distribution and recording all the various shapes. The furniture at the scene should not be used. If the scene has to be entered before the floor has been examined for shoeprints, plastic stepping slabs can be put onto the floor and walked on. These will scuff shoeprints but at least no other shoeprints will be added to the scene. The scene examiners and investigating officer must decide the best way to approach a scene to minimise disturbance. Any entry to the scene will cause disturbance. It is usual to photograph the scene at an early stage to provide a record so that any subsequent movements of furniture and so forth can be recognised. Sometimes furniture or other items are moved by a paramedic attempting resuscitation or by the person who found the body.

Only personnel authorised to be at a scene by the investigating officer should attend. Indeed, it is highly desirable, because of the need to limit access, to restrict the number of the scene team to a small but well-trained group of professionals.

According to one authority, the greatest problem he encountered in protecting the scene was the unauthorised attendance of police personnel and high-ranking officials coming along to help. This occurred particularly in the more 'high-profile' cases, which were attended by a great deal of publicity. They either contaminated or destroyed valuable evidence because they did not know what they were doing, or got in the way. They frequently left behind material, initially thought to be valuable trace evidence, which was consequently, needlessly examined. If the reader feels we are being a little unfair to senior police officers, it should be appreciated that these are the sentiments of a very experienced Lieutenent Commander of the New York City Police Department (Geberth, 1983).

SCENE ASSESSMENT – GENERAL APPROACH

Once the investigation team has been organised and a plan of action formulated, the detailed scene examination can begin. It is then important to define the scope of the scene. There may be other areas nearby that are involved. For example, there may have been a fight in a different area before the body was moved or dumped. There may be a weapon elsewhere. A person may have been observing the victim for some time and there may be some evidence at this spot to help identify the assailant. The team approach helps to ensure that all possible aspects are covered. A number of heads are often better than one in reading the scene to determine what may have happened. Each individual examiner must, however, be certain that they have checked it themselves and not rely on the possibility that another may have done so.

The only way to approach a scene examination is with a totally open mind. Any preconceived notions can adversely influence, consciously or otherwise, the efficiency of the investigation. There have been occasions when the scene examination of a murder was carried out perfunctorily as it was assumed to be a domestic offence. Later investigations showed that this initial assumption was not correct and, by then, it was impossible to recover the scene. The most obvious explanation of the murder may not be the correct one. For example, in a death by hypothermia the victim may shed or damage his clothing before death; blood at a scene may not relate to the present event; shoeprints may have been made sometime previously. Observation of the total scene may assist the examiner; for example, the state of the scene may indicate whether or not articles had been disturbed by the events, or whether they are in their normal position. The scene examiner is usually supplied with some information on the background to the offence. It is important to be sceptical about this; the information may be wrong or it may have been supplied by the person who will eventually become the suspect. During the course of the scene examination, more information may be gathered by the police investigating officers, which may change the original view of the event. If a suspect is arrested, the investigating officer will be very keen for the scene examiner to provide evidence from the scene to implicate him or her. The examiner must keep aloof from this and maintain a structured approach to the scene examination, while being aware of and sympathetic to the problems of the investigating officer. Obviously, the examiner must make sure that the investigating officer is kept up to date on the findings from the scene, which may change the direction of the investigation.

HEALTH HAZARDS, SAFETY AND SECURITY CONSIDERATIONS

There are many situations in which the site may be unsafe, especially after a conflagration. There may be noxious substances to consider, possible booby traps in explosion scenes, problems and difficulties with accessibility and dangerous terrain, etc. One must not overlook the risk, albeit slight, of infection by HIV and other microbial agents, which may be present in body fluids. Particular care should be taken in handling various surfaces and articles such as used and discarded hypodermic needles.

Each member of the team must safeguard themselves and other examiners. Some of the scientific methods used to recover or develop marks at a scene may be subject to COSSH Regulations (1988). If there are dangerous materials at a scene, the scene examiners may not be competent to deal with them. For example, a very badly burnt lady was found in a garage alongside a vat of liquid. The vat contained concentrated hydrochloric acid and a specialist chemical disposal team was brought in to dispose of this under the supervision of the investigating officer.

If one is dealing with a scene comprising premises that do not appear to be safe to enter, a surveyor should be called to assess safety. In scenes of terrorist offences, the area must be declared safe to enter by an expert in this type of scene; the possibility of booby traps should always be conisdered. One must also, in certain circumstances be aware of the possibility of contamination from radioactive substances, and advice from appropriate specialists should be sought prior to entry. Many scene examiners are civilians, and for protection and security a police attendance should be present at the scene.

In most indoor scenes, it is possible to wait until all dangers have been assessed and controlled with no loss of evidence. For outdoor scenes, however, it is more difficult to wait; a shoeprint may be washed away or fibres may be disturbed by the wind.

Illumination at a scene must be at least adequate. It is vital that the examiners are capable of seeing what is going on and what they are doing. Such a situation may arise particularly with outdoor scenes at night. Provision of appropriate illumination should be made and, indeed, nothing is lost in most cases by waiting till portable generators and lights are provided. For practical purposes, when a body is discovered at night, it is much more preferable to secure the scene and protect the body, by covering it with a tent, then to reconvene the investigation the next morning. Indeed, there is a very real risk of missing vital evidence when one is not working in daylight.

Lastly, there is the possibility of animals at the scene. Beware of cats and dogs who may not appreciate a scene examiner invading their domain. At least one scene examiner has been savaged by cats! Fleas and lice may also be a problem at a scene.

EXAMINATION OF THE BODY

Examination of the body at the scene may be carried out by a number of different investigators. Certification of the fact of death is usually carried out by the clinical forensic medical examiner (police surgeon) (see Chapter 3) or occasionally by the pathologist. The latter, however, usually arrives some time after the police have made their initial assessment of the scene and the body.

The purpose of examination of the body at the scene before transportation to the mortuary for autopsy is essentially fourfold:

1. Preliminary assessment where possible as to the type of death, i.e., whether it is a homicide, accident, suicide or due to natural causes.
2. To aid the investigation of a crime (if one has been committed) by collecting information, which leads to the arrest of a suspect and provides evidence against that person.
3. To collect such information about the body that will corroborate statements of witnesses and the suspect (where a crime is involved).
4. To maintain the integrity of the chain of custody of evidence.

RETROSPECTIVE SCENE VISIT

It should also be appreciated that the body may have been removed to hospital before, or soon after death, and hence cannot be viewed *in situ* at the scene. Nevertheless, much valuable information is frequently gained by a retrospective visit to the scene. Some would even argue that, on occasions, a visit after, rather than before, the post-mortem examination may be more beneficial to the pathologist, bearing in mind that he or she will have thoroughly assessed injuries and other significant marks at autopsy, and as a result be better placed to reconstruct events accurately leading to death and/or advise on the type of instrumentation causing trauma. In addition, there are occasions when, because of prevailing climatic conditions (as in the case described below) or poor lighting, it is necessary to return to the scene at a later stage, in some cases after the autopsy has been completed.

CASE 1.6

A night-watchman was found murdered within the hut of a building site. External bruises to his face and abdomen showed a well-defined circular configuration. The initial scene visit to the hut enabled assessment of where the incident actually happened to proceed in the usual manner. The search for a weapon, bearing in mind the findings of the pathologist, was delayed for a further two days, because the building site had become covered in a blanket of snow, after the deceased was killed and prior to his discovery. When the snow had melted, a piece of scaffolding pole was found, the end of which contained blood stains and matched the pattern of the wounds seen on the body.

References

Collinson J.G. (1970) The role of the investigating officer. *J. For. Sci. Soc.* **10**, 199–203.
COSSH (*Control of Substances Hazardous to Health, Control of Carcinogenic Substances*). HMSO, London, 1988.

Geberth V.J. (1983) *Practical Homicide Investigation.* Elsevier, New York.
Lewington F. (1990) *Scenes of Crime – Information for Police Officers. Biology Notes.* Metropolitan Police Forensic Science Laboratory, (copyright, Commissioner Metropolitan Police).
Zugibe F.T. and Costello J.T. (1993) The iceman murder: one of a series of contract murders. *J. For. Sci.* **38**, 1404–1408.

Further reading

Fisher B.A.J. (1993) *Techniques of Crime Scene Investigation*, 5th edn. CRC Press, Boca Raton, FL.

CHAPTER 2

Recording the scene

Recording or documentation of the scene must be carried out in a systematic way and carefully thought out prior to arrival at the scene. An accurate record is vital for the investigation and subsequent use as evidence in court. The body may be moved and objects shifted around at the scene; it is therefore essential that a full visual and written record is made from the moment the body is discovered. The endpoint of the scene record is sometimes difficult to gauge but most documentation is completed once the body has been removed to the mortuary, with further photographs taken, where appropriate, of the position where the body had been found.

Nowadays, with the advent of high technology, recording the scene is a great deal easier and more accurate than it used to be. More precise assessment is thus possible and recontruction of events more satisfactory.

Documentation of the scene

This comprises:

- Notes (written or dictated) and stills photography (the most essential elements of scene documentation).
- Video-recording, plans and sketches (frequently employed).
- Computer-aided packages and virtual reality (rarely used at present but have potential for future routine use).

Aids to scene recording

In addition to the photographer, other members of the scene team will require to make records of their attendance at the scene, which, indeed, may be used as evidence at a later date; it is important therefore to be well prepared. A number of aids may be used for such documentation, either for general use or for particular types of scenes. Body charts, templates with the outline of rooms, vehicles, etc. are always useful as an *aide-mémoire* for producing reports. Dictaphones, measuring instruments, instant picture cameras and portable video equipment, also have a role to play as tools that make note-taking more efficient.

The use of a dictaphone for note-taking at scenes has many advantages; the process is faster, notes tend to be more detailed and the problem of writing in wet conditions is avoided. If a voice-activated dictaphone is used then hands-free operation is possible; a considerable asset if the scene examiner is on a ladder or in any other position where safety demands that both hands be used to hold on. Where tape-recorded notes are made and subsequently transcribed, the transcript should be carefully checked against the original tape and then signed and dated as a true record of the original dictated notes. A word of caution needs to be added at this stage. Although recording onto tape at scenes is convenient, it is imperative to ensure that the dictaphone and batteries are in good working order. Secondly, the narrative should be checked before leaving the scene, in order to ensure that it has been satisfactorily recorded onto the tape. Nothing is worse than returning to one's office the next day to find that the tape does not contain some, or worse still, any of the information dictated into the recorder.

Measuring instruments vary from the simple to the extremely sophisticated (and expensive). Some form of tape measure is an essential piece of equipment. A surveyor's tape is ideal or, if the examiner is likely to work alone, then an ultrasonic measure may be more convenient. Used with care the latter can provide reasonably accurate measurements over distances up to 20 metres, although some instruments can be confused by intervening surfaces capable of reflecting the ultrasonic pulses.

Instant picture cameras and portable domestic video equipment are of great benefit in furnishing a record of the scene that can be viewed by other investigators and interested parties on the same day. It may be helpful to record evidence as it is discovered, particularly if there is a risk that the material might be damaged or obliterated by essential activities such as the making safe of hazardous structures. The quality of such photographs and recordings is variable and should only be used to supplement and not replace photographs, and video-recordings made to a professional standard.

Notes, sketches and plans

The preparation of scene notes and plans is an essential part of any scene examination (Figure 2.1(a), (b) and Figure 2.2). Firstly, they provide the examiner with an *aide-mémoire* when preparing statements or reports and, secondly, they document the actions taken at the scene. All the events appertaining to the scene should be documented in chronological order with the time recorded of each event or observation made. If they are to be used in a court of law, such notes should be contemporaneous, in other words, made while the matters in question are still fresh in the mind. Legal definitions of 'contemporaneous' do not specify any time limit but it is advisable for the scene examiner to complete the notes at the site, if at all possible, or as soon as possible thereafter on the same day. To avoid any confusion as to when they have been prepared, all hand-written notes and hand-drawn plans should be signed and dated, and any amendments or additions should be treated in a similar fashion. Such precautions are desirable in the light of the ever more common request in criminal courts that notes

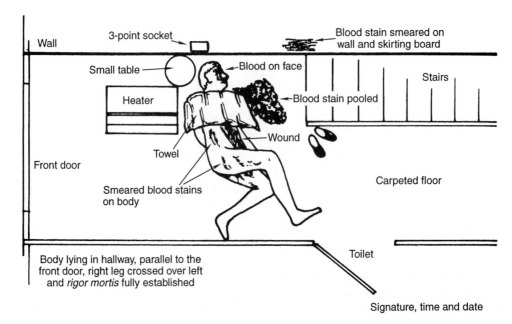

Wall

3-point socket

Blood stain smeared on wall and skirting board

Small table

Blood on face

Stairs

Heater

Blood stain pooled

Wound

Towel

Front door

Carpeted floor

Smeared blood stains on body

Body lying in hallway, parallel to the front door, right leg crossed over left and *rigor mortis* fully established

Toilet

Signature, time and date

Figure 2.1(a)   Sketch plan of the body *in situ* and the immediate environment.

be produced for scrutiny by counsel. Occasional use has also been made of scale models of crime scenes in murder trials in order to facilitate the presentation of a particularly complex case (Eckert, 1981; O'Brien, 1989).

'Stills' photography at the scene

The role of the scene of crime 'stills' photographer is to provide a high-quality permanent record of the scene, which will be essential for reference during the course of the investigation and ultimately be used as evidence in court (Scott, 1970). The photographer must at all times work harmoniously with the rest of the team, under the direction of the officer in charge of the scene. It is vitally important that the photographer has a standard procedure for documenting the scene from every angle, and at the same time ensuring that full account is taken of the specific needs of the officer in charge.

Priority should be given to ensure that there is no loss of evidential material, e.g., footwear impressions, before the photographer sets foot within the scene, and he or she may therefore have to be preceded by other specialists, in the interest of preserving such evidence.

The traditional practice of calling for the scene of crime officer and photographic support to attend immediately an incident is discovered is still in general use today and should be maintained. However, the trend these days is toward securing the scene of the incident without anyone impinging upon it until full discussion of the situation has been undertaken at a location nearby, such as a police station, formulating a detailed plan of action and convening appropriate personnel.

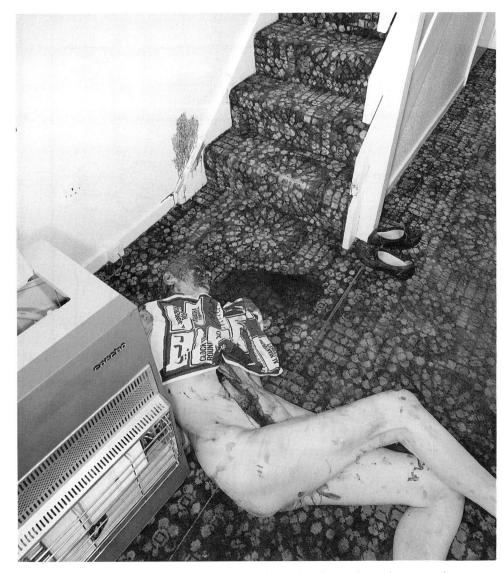

Figure 2.1(b)   A photograph of deceased. The sketch was drawn from a similar viewpoint.

Scene contamination is obviously an extremely important consideration. The photographer needs to take care where the photographic equipment is placed whilst working. Space can be improvised at a scene, which has been forensically cleared, so that equipment can be laid out for easy access. Whilst at the scene, accurate records should be kept in the form of contemporaneous notes of the photographer's attendance, and subsequent important events, such as body removal, fingerprint and footprint photography for future production in court, if necessary.

If the scene is to be video-recorded, it is important for the stills photographer to work

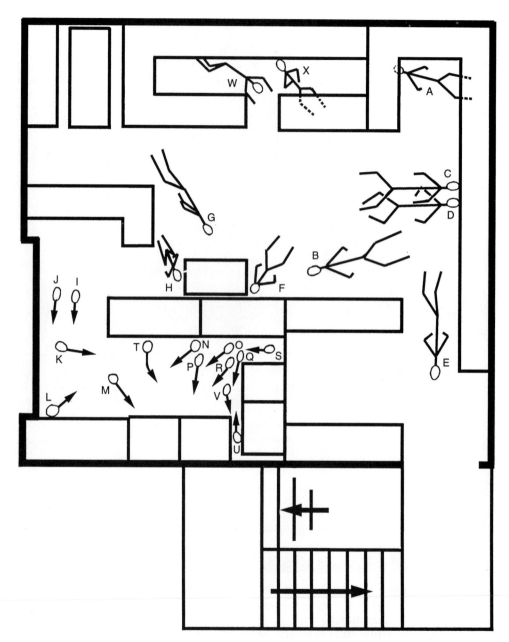

Figure 2.2 A plan of a multiple death scene from a fire. The position and unique identifying label of each body is shown, thus allowing one to check the location of each body after recovery.

closely with the video team so as to provide an accurate and balanced visual documentation of the scene. Broadly the 'stills' person should concentrate on photography that will be studied in detail by the investigating team, whilst the video team should expect to cover the whole scene from top to bottom, showing the position of various objects, in relation to one another.

For example, a video camera could cover a typical room, starting from the doorway, and traversing the room in a clockwise direction, then record walls, ceiling, floor, furniture and the deceased in good detail, and conclude the operation in about 15 minutes. On the other hand, the 'stills' photographer, in order to cover the same scene, might take 20 or 30 photographs over a period of several hours.

On arrival at the scene, the first objective of the photographer is to find the senior officer dealing with the case or the deputy, and also to establish a close working relationship with the scene of crime officer, with whom most of the filming will be done. For the photographer it is of great importance to know as much as is currently known by the officer in the case concerning the incident, as it will dictate how he or she is to operate. The photographer will then be able, with the scene of crime officer, to approach the scene using the best 'agreed route' to avoid contaminating or disturbing evidence in any way.

Having ascertained clearance and wearing the necessary protective overclothing, the 'stills' photographer will record the scene, starting from immediately outside the premises concerned, showing points of entry such as the front door, or passageway, observing and avoiding disturbance to any blood-splashing, damage to doors and walls, footwear marks, hand-smears, visible fingerprints etc., which will need subsequent photography in detail by the investigating team.

In the case of a public house or club incident, it is essential that before any vehicles outside the premises are allowed to leave, drivers within the immediate vicinity are recorded on video to show their exact positions together with the registration plates of their cars.

The photographer will then work slowly through the scene in conjunction with scene of crime officers, toward the area containing the deceased, vacating the scene from time to time, to allow thorough video-recording of the location. The latter will be expected to cover the position of various objects within the scene, and potential escape and entry routes, and any other aspect of the scene as necessary. Although differing circumstances may dictate the best approach in each scene, the photographer must be mindful of the fact that it is essential in all cases to record the evidence *in situ*, before it is examined or disturbed in any way.

When the photographer finally arrives at the area containing the deceased, it is necessary to take several photographs of the immediate surroundings, before moving closer to photograph the body in greater detail. Before photography commences, it is important to ascertain from the other scene visitors, the original position of objects and whether they have been moved, taken away or have been added after the deceased was found. The same holds true for the position of clothing of the deceased and adjacent potential murder weapon. The photographer should use his or her experience, together with that of the officer in charge of the case, and should take special care, preferably by using close-up photography, to document articles on or near the deceased that may have relevance to the crime, such as keys, money, letters, other objects, marks, visible injuries to the deceased, damage to clothing, etc., in a more detailed manner.

All these items should be recorded in sufficient detail, in order to enable accurate comparisons with subsequent photography undertaken in the mortuary or laboratory, so that there is no question as to their authenticity.

Turning to the photographic equipment that can be used, there is no such thing as the ideal 'scene of crime' camera, and photographers must be fully aware of the requirements of the work they are undertaking, and have available the most appropriate and versatile equipment, in order to achieve the highest possible standard of documentation. As different forces have different budgets, work loads, and other constraints, it is not surprising that a variety of equipment and film formats exist at different levels.

The Metropolitan Police in London, for example, for a number of years have used the Pentax and Bronica GS-1, 6 × 7 systems, with wide-angle and macro lenses fitted to both. The standard lens, although supplied with each kit, is used mainly in an outdoor mode to produce photographs of a scene or location with angle of view equated to that of the human eye. Bearing in mind that almost all interiors, and certainly sites of arsons, and scenes occurring after dark, will require supplementary lighting of some kind, flash units, such as the Metz Mecablitz 60 and CT#5 are used, and where a second flash is required, this is fired by a slave unit, held conveniently by a scene officer.

When all the photography concerning the location and the deceased have been concluded, and the body removed, the next stage of photography is undertaken. This usually consists of recording in colour, and black and white such items as shoe marks or impressions (in either blood, earth or even in snow), inside or outside the premises. The pattern of blood spattering and pooling, should be thoroughly documented. Blood spatter, footwear impressions and other marks (tool marks and fingerprints) will need to be photographed with a 90° angle scale placed next to the subject, for eventual reproduction to the same size. Specialised equipment may be used for this purpose. Similarly, bullet holes, shot-gun pellet spread, and weapon damage within the scene, should be recorded with a scale, complementing the overall picture gained by the video team.

It is sometimes beneficial to the enquiry to take photographs from a high vantage point overlooking the scene, to illustrate the position of witnesses, vehicles, etc. If a tall block of flats or similar vantage point cannot be used, then a helicopter or light aircraft could provide the required assistance. No special equipment is necessary to obtain high-quality photographs from the air, and many examples of scene of crime work exist where a Pentax or Bronica have been used.

Once the first phase of photography at a scene of crime has been completed, the officer in charge of the case may request, in due course, the attendance of specialists who have the facility to record marks and impressions at the scene, which are invisible to the naked eye. Such techniques often require the scene to be darkened, so that high-intensity ultraviolet light sources or a portable laser may be used (see Chapter 5). These light sources cause various substances to fluoresce in different ways, and the appropriate photographic film, lens and exposures would have to be used to record these findings.

Video-recording at the scene

Over the years, the method that we believe gives the best all-round results in any serious incidents, such as homicides, suspicious deaths and in major disasters, is for the 'stills' photographer who has developed the necessary skills to operate a video camera, to be assigned to video the scene. He or she preferably does this on a single-handed basis, and it is his or her sole responsibility to duplicate, document and present for court purposes any video evidence that appertains to an individual case.

In the Metropolitan Police, the video photographer is supplied with a vehicle, specially fitted out with the electronic facility to transfer the recording which is formatted originally on high-band m.II. to VHS. This master tape format is full broadcast quality. The copy facility can be powered from either 240 volt mains supply or from internally fitted batteries. The vehicle is also fitted with an external light source, which can be powered from a variety of sources, including an on-board generator and allows illumination of an external scene. Suitable recommended camera systems included the Sony DXC 3000 (fitted with an ultra-wide angle zoom ranging from 6 mm up to 96 mm) coupled to a Sony video cassette recorder or the Panasonic M2 system.

Although most video teams consist of two or more operators, the ability to use only a single person at the scene of a crime has the advantage that, when suitably gowned and wearing protective overshoes, scene disturbance is kept to an absolute minimum. It does however mean that the camera operator has to carry all the equipment for the duration of the recording. This will consist of camcorder (camera and recorder), spare batteries, spare tapes, portable light and its power source (either a camera-mounted battery or a battery belt). The approximate total weight of this equipment adds up to 20 kg.

Although it is preferable to use the video camera on a tripod whenever possible for maximum stability and quality, the camera operator must have mobility in a confined area, and be capable of zooming and changing focus during filming, whilst still holding the camera steady (especially when filming close-ups). The video camera will normally be fitted with a small artificial light source placed directly over the lens, so that a shadowless illumination of the scene may be obtained. This light should be capable of running from a portable source (probably a 30-volt battery belt or a camera mounted 12-volt battery) and be able to provide a minimum duration of about 20–30 minutes (using an increased gain setting on the camera, if necessary).

Despite the versatile nature of video-recording, it should nevertheless be appreciated that, for best definition and detail, the 'stills' photographer is as yet unsurpassed in being able to produce images of the highest possible quality.

Special care must be taken to record such items as:

- Doors and windows, to show whether they are open or closed, or have been forced.
- Televisions and radios, to show whether they are switched on or off, and to identify to which channels they are tuned.
- Items of clothing, and accessories such as shoes, jewellery and handbags.
- Items bearing writing or labelling, and any books, diaries and similar objects.
- Other items, which reveal aspects of the person's habits and occupation.
- Containers of food, drink or medication showing evidence of socio-economic conditions, including evidence of neglect.

You have only one chance to record the scene in pristine condition and, as video tape is probably the cheapest part of the equipment, it makes sense to be thorough. One never knows what facts may come to light, days or even months later, that the recording may verify or negate.

Once the body has been reached via a previously cleared and approved route, a complete coverage of the body and its position is necessary, showing clothing, injuries, blood marks, exposed parts of the body, usually hands and face, and, where possible, the presence and distribution of hypostasis, although a complete photographic documentation of the deceased will be carried out in the mortuary.

It is obviously necessary to obtain more than one aspect or view of the deceased, especially the injuries or main points of interest, which may not be immediately visible. The scene of crime officer must therefore clear a second path round the deceased so that an alternative viewpoint may be obtained. Whilst this is being done, other aspects of the investigation are continuing; the 'stills' photographer can be photographing the body, weapons, blood splashes, etc. and the video cameraman can cover approach routes, blood trails and debris from the incident such as broken bottles.

On returning to the deceased, the body can be recorded from a variety of angles, again including injuries, weapon and blood splashes, and their direction, in as great a detail as possible. Once the area has been forensically examined and clearance given, the video camera operator should cover all other rooms in the building, especially those that give access to the main part of the scene, such as the hallways and stairs. This should be done whether or not they have any apparent bearing on the investigation, because it may be several days later before any link can be established and then the rooms may well have been disturbed by police search teams. Once again, particular attention must be paid to all items of property on tables, mantlepieces, bookshelves and on the floor. It is good practice, not only to record the tops of desks, tables, etc., to show the letters, notepads and any pieces of paper present, but also to include in large close-up, any information contained which may be relevant so that, for future reference, their exact placing can be shown. Such detailed documentation should enable any allegations concerning the introduction of incriminating evidence to be refuted.

Any movement of the body by police officers during the initial examination, either to ascertain the presence of further injuries, the cause of death, or examination of the contents of the deceased's clothing, must be recorded on video with, if possible, the camera placed on a tripod. Close liaison with the scene of crime officer and the senior fingerprint officer is essential at this point so that no evidence is accidentally destroyed or remains unrecorded, and no opportunity is given to the defence to allege malpractice or doubt of any kind.

The pathologist may or may not be present during the initial scene examination carried out by the scene of crime officer, but if he or she is present, any suggestions he or she may make concerning the body, its injuries or position, should be recorded for future reference.

It is always good practice to warn all those in the vicinity of the video-recorder, especially when sound is also being recorded, that the microphone used on these occasions will pick up any conversation over a very wide area.

When it is deemed appropriate for the deceased to be removed, it may be necessary to record the process of moving the body onto the body sheet in preparation for 'bagging up', in case some previously hidden object is revealed. It can then be shown to have always been present. Once the body has left the scene, another recording should be made of the area immediately beneath it to show the condition of the surface, which may be affected by body fluids. Furthermore, it is good practice for the photographer and video camera operator to remain behind until the officer in charge is satisfied that all aspects of the scene have been recorded to his or her satisfaction.

At the conclusion of the filming at the scene, the master tapes are taken back to the video control van where a complete copy can be made at the scene. This has the advantage that a VHS copy can be presented to the investigating officer almost immediately. This can be played back at the scene or viewed subsequently by officers, thereby reducing the need for them all to attend the scene of the incident. There is also the benefit that, over the first few hours or days of the enquiry, the investigating officer can refer to any points arising from developments by viewing the tape, without waiting for the album of colour photographs, which may take longer to arrive.

Once the incident has progressed to the point where a person is charged with the offence, it will be necessary to make a court copy from the master tapes. This copy is supplied on the U-Matic format so that the best-quality evidence may be viewed in court without risking damage to the original tape.

Plan drawing

COMPUTERISED SCENE RECORDING

In recent years, a number of computerised aids to scene recording have become available. These are either site survey packages or portable plan drawing systems. Site survey equipment is generally a combination of a direction and range recording instrument coupled to a robust portable computer running an appropriate software package. Most of the systems available are capable of downloading data in a suitable format for use in computer-aided design (CAD) systems incorporating high-quality large-format plotters.

Examples of the systems currently available include the GRiD Systems Corporation GRiDPAD™, a robust portable computer, which has an LCD touch screen and pen-based input. Current models use an internal modem to facilitate transfer of data to other microcomputers. Storage options include hard discs and memory cards, though the latter require a card interface on a receiving machine. The use of a pen-based input does away with the need for the most vulnerable part of the computer, a keyboard, out at the scene but this may have disadvantages in that some software may not be able to run on the system without modification.

Hardware that can be connected to a portable computer, which includes the Carl Zeiss Total Station™, an electronic theodolite, can accurately measure positions from a datum point. Its range makes it suitable for outdoor scenes spread over large areas. The use of software adapted from an archaeological package allows the survey and logging of extended sites, such as vehicle accidents and explosions.

Photogrammetry is a further technique in which computers may assist in scene recording. Strictly, this is an aid for the preparation of plans after the incident but it requires some work at the scene. If scene photographs are taken with a three-axis scale in them it is possible to derive the true dimensions of many objects in the photograph by careful measurement. This is an extremely time-consuming process if carried out manually, and its accuracy is dependent upon there being no distortion of the scene by the camera. Computer systems exist that can take stereoscopic photo pairs or even ordinary photographs, and draw up scale plans from them. The main disadvantages of these systems are that they are extremely expensive at present and can only show what can be seen in the photographs.

In assessing whether photogrammetry is worthwhile, the value of locating objects exactly at the scene and the ability to prepare high-quality plans of scenes must be weighed against the cost of the equipment, and the expense of training people to use it effectively. In many instances the amount of use to which such equipment will be put is the deciding factor.

THE FUTURE – 'VIRTUAL REALITY'

One extension of the use of computerised plans is into the field of virtual reality (VR), which uses a computer model to generate three-dimensional images, allowing a subject to 'walk through' a scene. The systems currently available can be either desktop based, using computers and monitors, or 'immersion' systems where the viewer wears a headset that gives the illusion of being within the environment being displayed.

In a forensic context, the investigator could examine the reconstruction of an incident, using it to obtain and evaluate witness evidence and, in the case of vehicle accidents or fires, it might be possible to model the progress of the incident and test various scenarios. VR is presently being used in fire service training programmes to demonstrate fire modelling, escape theory and human behaviour, and to visualise fire and egress scenarios (Anon., 1994).

Widespread forensic use of VR would almost certainly have to rely upon the computerised recording of the scene and the routine provision of display equipment in the courts. The low cost and ready availability of desktop video displays means that they are likely to appear in courts some time before immersion systems, but the expense of preparing the computer models will probably limit the use of VR at first to major enquiries and proceedings involving serious crime.

Despite being in the experimental stage, the introduction of such techniques is inevitable but the use of the technology will have to be accompanied by safeguards. VR-based evidence in criminal proceedings could be misused or abused; the tendency of people to believe what they see raises the possibility that juries will be swayed by computerised models and reconstructions which reflect prejudices of those who develop them. In adversarial proceedings VR may well be introduced to bolster a version of reality favourable to the commisioning party's case. The failure of a jury to appreciate that the 'reality' in VR is nothing of the sort could lead to miscarriages of justice.

References

Anon. (1994) Fire Service College uses Virtual Reality. *Health Safety Indust. Commerce* **17**, 4.
Eckert W.G. (1981) Miniature crime scenes. *Am. J. For. Med. Path.* **2**, 365–368.
O'Brien M.W. (1989) Scale model use in crime trials. *J. For. Ident.* **39**, 359–366.
Scott H. (1970) The role of the photographer. *J. For. Sci. Soc.* **10**, 205–212.

Further reading

Redsicker D.R. (1991) *The Practical Methodology of Forensic Photography.* Elsevier, New York.

CHAPTER 3

The forensic pathologist and other medical personnel at the scene

There appears to be a wide regional variation in the frequency of attendance at a scene by a pathologist, depending on local practice and to some extent on the volume of casework. In some areas the pathologist will be expected to go to all scenes whenever requested to do so by the local constabulary. In other regions, attendance is not obligatory but is rather at the discretion of the investigating officer, in consultation with the pathologist. It is under the latter circumstances that there is always the possible risk of evidence crucial to the investigation being lost or misinterpreted, if the pathologist does not attend. Visiting every scene may not be practicable, but one should not underestimate the wealth of invaluable information and experience that may be gained by regular attendance. Indeed, even if the body has been removed to the mortuary, every effort should be made to allow the pathologist full access to the scene. When a pathologist is attempting to reconstruct the chain of events leading to death, an awareness of the scene of the fatal incident, the objects within such a scene, the type of location and so on, may help to explain, for example, minor injuries that are found, as well as the more obvious major fatal wounds.

In a substantial number of cases, as in the following example, a scene visit followed promptly by a post-mortem examination to ascertain whether or not foul play is involved, enables the investigating officer to make an appropriate early decision regarding deployment of manpower, and thus keep the cost of the investigation to a minimum.

CASE 3.1

A 55-year-old male who lived alone in a flat had not been seen for a week. A worried friend informed the police, who found him in his premises after they had forced an entry. His living room was in a state of disarray and he was lying virtually naked in a prone position. Clearly the appearance of the scene and the multiple superficial injuries on the body gave rise to a suspicion of foul play. An autopsy was carried out the same evening, within three hours of the pathologist's visit to the scene and revealed that he had died from bacterial meningitis (Figure 3.1(a) and (b)).

The pathologist should therefore take into account the following when visiting the scene:

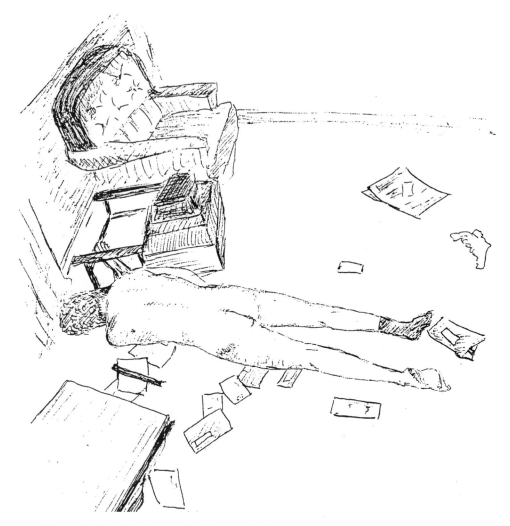

Figure 3.1(a)   The deceased is shown naked and face down. Furniture in the room had been knocked over and there were items of correspondence scattered over the floor. A few scattered bruises can also be seen on the body.

1. The environment.
2. The condition and position of the body at the locus, also taking into account attempts at resuscitation.
3. Consideration of the circumstances surrounding death in relation to the body and the scene.
4. Interpretation of post-mortem findings in the light of scene examination.

In order to avoid omitting any important elements of the scene examination, it is wise to adopt a systematic approach to the task in hand such as the following.

1. Preparation. The pathologist should ensure that he or she has a dictaphone, notepaper, writing implements and a rectal thermometer. Body charts, pen torch and a small ruler are also useful and can be easily carried on one's person.

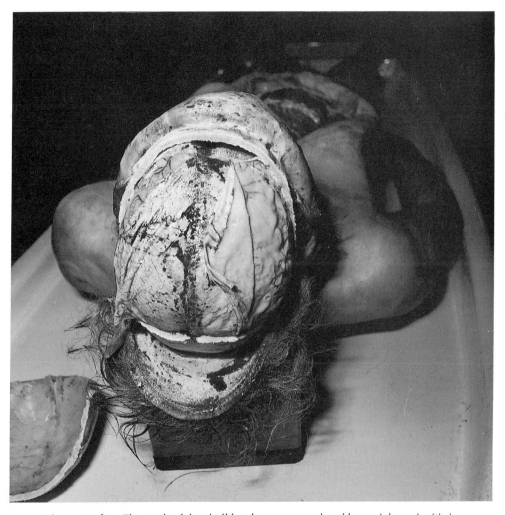

Figure 3.1(b)   The vault of the skull has been removed and bacterial meningitis is evident.

2. Record the time requested to attend the scene and the name and status of the person making the request. Custom will vary within different medico-legal systems as to the person contacting the pathologist. In Scotland, the pathologist is contacted by a procurator fiscal, whereas in England and Wales, it may either be a coroner's officer or senior police officer.
3. On arrival at the scene, the pathologist should in all circumstances report to the officer at the entrance to the scene in order that the time of his or her arrival and identity can be recorded.
4. He or she should then don protective clothing and wait to be guided to the body via the agreed route of access. At this stage the chief scene investigator or one of his or her colleagues should be available to describe the circumstances of the discovery of the body.

5.   The pathologist should then ascertain from the senior investigating officer what is required of him or her. Under no circumstances should the pathologist go straight to the body and start examining it without leave to do so. There are many reasons for this, contamination of the scene and irredeemable loss of trace evidence being the two principal ones. Adequate lighting, e.g., from a portable generator, will ensure that such errors are not made.

6.   The body should then be described as found *in situ*, together with its immediate environment including its posture, clothing and relationship to the other objects in its immediate vicinity.

7.   Examination of the body for the purposes of preliminary assessment of marks and/or injuries to the body.

8.   Time of death assessment, if appropriate.

9.   Advise the scene investigators on the protection of trace evidence on the body during transportation to the mortuary.

10.   Provide a description of other areas near the body, e.g., other rooms in the house.

11.   Supervise removal of the body from the scene.

In addition to the above, care must be taken when attending the scene to avoid:

1.   Giving 'off the cuff' and premature views to investigating officers.

2.   Being influenced by senior investigating officers into assuming death has occurred in a certain manner, particularly when all the relevant facts surrounding the case are not yet to hand and examination of the body is incomplete.

3.   Having any contact with members of the mass media. Frequently newspaper and television reporters, and camera operators are present around the scene, hoping for any snippets of information, particularly if the case is likely to generate a great deal of public interest. Occasionally they will go to extraordinary lengths to take photographs of the scene or monitor conversations between people. The pathologist should therefore be cognisant of the strictly confidential nature of the enquiries and the need to adopt a cautious attitude throughout the visit. If a press conference is to be arranged, this is the responsibility of the chief scene investigator through the appropriate press liaison officer.

Arrival and preliminary assessment

On arrival at a scene, the pathologist will find that part of the area in question will have been protected in some way from persons not entitled to be there for obvious reasons of contamination. He or she will be asked his or her name, and this will be recorded, together with the time of arrival, by a police officer at the entrance to the scene. The pathologist may have been thoroughly briefed beforehand regarding the circumstances but, in any case, should be fully appraised on arrival. In complex and multiple suspicious deaths, the forensic team, including the pathologist, should have conferred to draw up a plan of action before detailed examination begins. In most situations, however, the pathologist's knowledge of the circumstances is limited prior to his or her arrival at the scene and he or she will rely very much on the guidance given by the investigating officer. Indeed, it is essential that before beginning his or her examination he or she seeks the advice of the investigating officer and/or the scene of crime officer. He or she will then be in a position to know to what extent the body should be examined *in situ*, where in the environment access is allowed to, the agreed route by which to approach the body and what he or she is allowed to touch. It must be borne in mind that other scientists and police officers will need to examine the scene in detail for the collection and recording of evidence, and this must always be in the forefront of the pathologist's mind. At this point the pathologist should enquire whether photographs of the body and the scene have been taken, and should direct the photographer to take specific and close views of the body as necessary.

Examination of the body and its environment

Examination of the body, its position, condition (state of preservation), distribution of injuries, etc., should be carried out in conjunction with a description of the scene and not in isolation.

As discussed in Chapter 1, it is necessary to appreciate that where the body is discovered may not be where death occurred. It is essential therefore to establish what the scene of discovery of the body represents. Is it where death occurred or was the deceased transported there from elsewhere, for example? By careful examination of the body at its location there may be obvious signs that the body has been transported in some way. There may be binding of hands and feet to facilitate this, there may be drag marks, clothing on the body inappropriate for the scene of discovery, evidence of storage in one particular environment for some time before transportation to another type and so on. It may be necessary, where appropriate, for the pathologist to visit other related 'scenes'.

The investigating officer may be able to give the pathologist a comprehensive account of the circumstances leading to death and the pathologist should always be satisfied that his or her examination supports the account given.

One of the first things that a pathologist may be asked to ascertain at the scene, is whether or not foul play had occurred. He or she may feel able, for example, to say with confidence that the death was due to natural causes and thus curtail a potentially expensive homicide investigation. In practice, however, in the majority of suspicious deaths, this is not resolved until the autopsy is carried out. In such cases, where the situation is not clear either way, one should expedite the post-mortem examination and ensure that, meanwhile, the scene is fully secured and undisturbed.

It is usually difficult to examine the body externally in a comprehensive manner at the scene and indeed there is no point in attempting to do so. The body, which may be clothed, is usually not undressed until its arrival at the mortuary and then only by the pathologist, or under his or her direction. If it is felt, however, that movement of the clothed body may cause contamination of the clothing, e.g. from blood emanating from stab wounds, then the removal of the clothing is justified, provided the pathologist is fully aware of the type and distribution of such clothing on the body, and is able to examine it fully. This procedure should be documented fully and carried out carefully to avoid loss of trace evidence. This should only be done when absolutely essential. The distribution, state and type of visible clothing should be noted.

The position of the body, the distribution of rigor mortis and the position of hypostasis, where possible, should also be noted. Minimal disturbance should be the aim of the pathologist at this stage. The main part of the external examination is much better left until the post-mortem examination is carried out in the mortuary.

The following two cases illustrate a number of important aspects of scene examination discussed above.

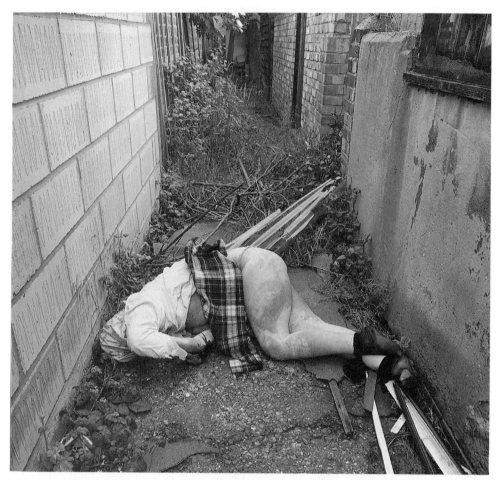

Figure 3.2(a)   The victim is shown lying face down as found in an alley behind a row of terraced houses. Her clothes were dishevelled, her head covered with a plastic shopping bag, and her hands and feet had been bound.

CASE 3.2

A 12-year-old girl failed to return home from school. Twenty-four hours later her body was found in an alley behind a row of terraced houses (Figure 3.2(a)). She lived in one of the houses in the same street. One of the initial problems addressed was whether or not she was killed at the scene where she was found. As one can see from Figure 3.2(b) and (c), the body had been in a cramped position (doubled up) inside a confined space for a number of hours before being transported to the scene. This is evident from the distribution and demarcation of the hypostasis and the pressure marks on the knees. The hands and feet were bound so as to facilitate transportation of the body, and a plastic carrier bag had been placed over her head and secured with adhesive tape to prevent spillage of blood during transportation. In addition, the scene had restricted access and great care had to be taken when walking towards the body so as not to

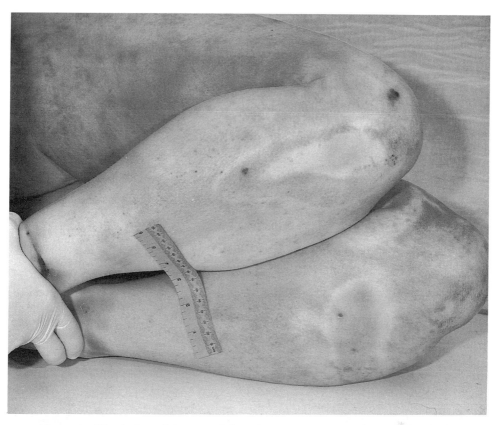

Figure 3.2(b)   A view of the victim's legs showing pressure marks just below both knees where they had been pressed against the inside of a car boot in a flexed position similar to that shown in the photograph.

interfere with any physical evidence such as potential shoeprints. There was minimal handling of clothing in this case because of the need for examination by the Serious Crime Unit (Chapter 4).

CASE 3.3

The body of a young adult female, found about 50 metres from a motorway in a field behind some trees, had been concealed by placing a white sheet and various other items over her which had been found at the location. On removing these it was noted that the deceased had had her clothing shifted from its normal position because she had been held and dragged to where she was found. Her lower back and buttocks were covered with soil and vegetation, as was the clothing. Furthermore, there were quite clear drag marks to the backs of both legs as well as to the buttocks, indicating that she had been held by her arms and dragged backwards (Figure 3.3(a) and (b)). It was established at the autopsy that she had been strangled, and it later transpired that her boyfriend had killed her at her home and transported her body by car 40 km, to the place where she was discovered.

Examination of the immediate environment (where the body is lying) is essential

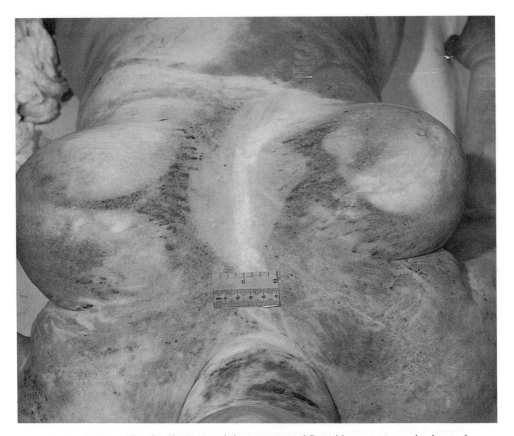

Figure 3.2(c) The distribution and demarcation of florrid hypostasis on the front of the chest and abdomen clearly indicates how she had been in a cramped postion and the body 'doubled up' for a number of hours in a confined space.

and will help the pathologist to have a better understanding of the events leading to death. There may be pooling of blood, which can be matched later with injuries, vomited material and other body substances, such as saliva, urine, faeces, etc., which by their position and quantity may be of assistance to the pathologist in his investigation. The type and extent of damage to furniture or structures within a room may assist in reconstructing the various positions and movement of persons at a scene during a fatal attack, particularly when related to the distribution of injuries on the body.

At this stage the investigating officer may need some guidance as to the post-mortem interval (time of death) and this is discussed below.

A general examination of the scene by the pathologist may be valuable, particularly if areas of disturbance, blood, etc., are found away from the body, for example, in other locations in a house. It may be necessary to give explanations for some injuries found, which may, for example, fit with falling down a flight of stairs even though the deceased may have been found in the sitting room.

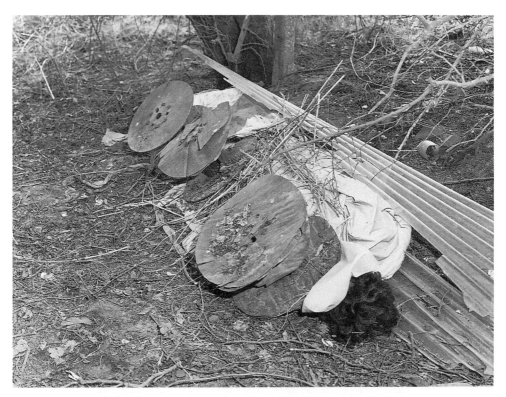

Figure 3.3(a)   The deceased is shown *in situ* in a field near a tree and by some bushes. She is face down, and had been covered by a number of items, and hidden from view from the nearby motorway.

Ascertaining the fact of death

When a body is discovered, the initial action is to ascertain whether or not the person found at the scene is in fact dead. Anyone can presume death but only a medically qualified practitioner should certify the fact of death according to standard, though not statutory, practice, even though this may be plainly obvious. Usually, it is the clinical forensic medical examiner (police surgeon) who is called to the scene to carry out such an examination and, indeed, he or she may also be in a position to give some guidance as to the nature of the death (whether suspicious or otherwise). Strictly speaking, however, once death has been ascertained, the involvement of the forensic medical examiner ends and the pathologist should then be called if the death is thought to be suspicious. Occasionally, where it is more expedient, the pathologist may be asked to certify death.

Care must taken in certain cases to ensure that erroneous diagnosis of the fact of death is not made, particularly when dealing with conditions known to be associated with so called 'suspended animation', such as hypothermia or certain types of drug overdoses, most notably barbiturates. Mullan et al. (1965) described two cases of

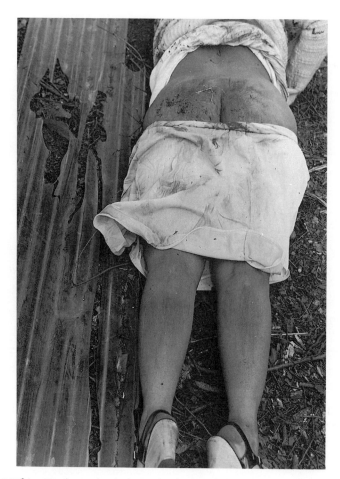

Figure 3.3(b)   Her lower back, buttocks, legs and clothing are contaminated with soil and vegetation. Drag marks are also present and are particularly obvious on the backs of both legs. Because of dragging by the arms, her upper clothing has ridden up and the skirt rolled down.

barbiturate poisoning in patients who had been certified dead by a medical practitioner, but who were subsequently found to be alive.

There are numerous other cases reported in the press and cited in standard texts, including the case of a young woman of 23 years, described by Polson et al. (1985). She was found on a beach near Liverpool by two lorry drivers who summoned a local doctor. He reported that the body appeared to him to be dead and a pathologist who arrived later at the scene agreed with this view. When the body was taken to the mortuary, however, and the post-mortem was due to begin, one of the persons present noticed an eyelid flickering and the formation of a tear. She was promptly covered with clothing and sent to the intensive care unit, and eventually went on to make a full recovery.

Assessing the post-mortem interval (time of death)

In a substantial number of cases, the question of the post-mortem interval, i.e., the period elapsed between death and discovery of the body, comes into question and the investigating officer may need some guidance.

The following factors may be taken into account at the scene:

- Cooling of the body.
- Rigor mortis.
- Hypostasis.
- Putrefactive changes.
- Infestation by insects.

A core body temperature (usually rectal) should be taken at the scene where feasible and deemed safe to do so by the investigating officer. Alternatively, if the scene conditions are not condusive (they may be ill-lit, cramped, wet, etc.), it is better to take the temperature in the mortuary. The pathologist may use either a mercury-in-glass thermometer with a range of 0–100 °C, or a thermometer that works on the principle of the thermocouple giving a digital read-out with an accuracy of about 0.1 °C.

Before taking a core reading at the scene, move any clothing present carefully to one side or remove the garments (avoid cutting off clothing), to allow the standard swabs (anal and rectal in all cases) to be taken prior to the introduction of a thermometer into the rectum. In females, external and internal vaginal swabs should also be taken because of the possibility of contamination by the introduction and removal of a thermometer (particularly in a cramped and possibly ill-lit environment).

The environmental temperature should be taken quite close to the body and should ideally be taken as early as possible after discovery of the body. This can be carried out by a police officer or scenes of crime officer. It is especially important when dealing with a body in an enclosed environment, such as a room, to take the temperature before it is filled with people, or the window opened, or heating turned off (all these factors may change the environmental temperature by several degrees). The heating conditions, and particularly in modern centrally heated houses, the times at which the heating is set to come on and off, should all be taken into account.

With an outdoor scene, the temperature change is usually much more variable and unpredicatable, particularly in the British Isles. Windy conditions and rain, for example, may have prevailed between death and discovery of the body, making any useful assessment very difficult. Meteorological records may assist.

Preliminary assessment of rigor mortis should be made at the scene and more thoroughly and systematically at the mortuary. Hypostasis, however, particularly if the body is clothed, is better assessed at the mortuary. Its distribution is sometimes of use in indicating whether a body had previously been in a different position for at least a large number of hours or days.

Putrefactive changes generally only allow one to make an approximate assessment of the post-mortem interval in relation to the environment in which the body is found. The presence of insects and other invertebrates, which are concomitant with such changes, may help enormously in this respect (see Chapter 6).

For detailed guidance on time of death estimation in relation to the above parameters (excluding entomological methods), the reader may wish to consult Knight (1995).

Artefacts due to resuscitation attempts

First aid and, occasionally, major surgery may have been carried out at the scene, and one must always bear this in mind. In attempting to save life, the doctors or paramedics are not going to concern themselves with the need to preserve trace evidence, or worry whether their thoracotomy incision is going to modify or incorporate a particular wound. Their thoughts will be directed solely to saving the victim's life. Consequently, when life is deemed to be extinct and the medical team have left the scene, it is inevitable that they will have altered the body and the scene to a certain extent. The pathologist should therefore be made aware that resuscitation attempts have been carried out so that any resulting artefacts (such as the examples given below) may be given due consideration during the course of the investigation. The resuscitation team should be questioned as to what they found initially and what they did.

   The following are examples of how the body and the scene may be altered as a result of resuscitation.

1.   New wounds may be formed to effect drainage of cavities, particularly on the chest, which may resemble stab wounds. If examined at the scene in relation to any blood pattern, erroneous conclusions may be drawn.
2.   A stab wound may, on occasions, have a drain inserted in it and initially may not be thought of as significant.
3.   A surgeon frequently incorporates a stab wound into a thoracotomy or laparotomy incision, and the injury may therefore not be immediately apparent at the scene.
4.   Wounds resulting from placing drips, either punctures or 'cut down' wounds, are common and need to be differentiated from needle punctures in the arms due to recent intravenous drug abuse.
5.   The position of the body is frequently substantially shifted from its original position and may also have been turned over.
6.   Foreign bodies may have been left in a body cavity or in the air passages.
7.   Surfaces may be smeared with transferred blood or other fluids from the body by medical personnel.
8.   Extraneous material may be left behind by the medical team such as syringes, packaging, etc.

Removal of the body from the scene

The pathologist should be available to supervise the removal of the body from a scene, and circumvent and assist with the interpretation of any potential post-mortem injuries that may occur in the unlikely event of dropping the body, or indeed, through clumsy handling.

   The body should always be bagged before removal to the mortuary. This includes the application of protective waterproof bags to the head, hands and feet. At this stage, the pathologist should enquire that the appropriate trace evidence has been collected from the exposed parts of the body. It should be borne in mind that the integrity of the chain of evidence must be maintained fully and that the body is accompanied by a police officer to the mortuary.

References

Knight B. (ed.) (1995) *The Estimation of the Time since Death in the Early Postmortem Period.* Edward Arnold, London.

Mullan D., Platts M. and Ridgeway B. (1965) Barbiturate intoxication. *Lancet* **1**, 705.

Polson C.J., Gee D.J. and Knight B. (1985) *The Essentials of Forensic Medicine*, 4th edn. Pergamon, Oxford, pp.3–4.

Usher A. (1970) The role of the pathologist at the scene of crime. *J. For. Sci. Soc.* **10**, 213–218.

CHAPTER 4

The forensic scientist and scene of crime officer at the scene

Locard's principle

The fundamental guiding principle that underlies the approach to any scene examination is attributable to Edmond Locard. The latter was head of the Institute of Criminalistics in the University of Lyon in France and produced his *Manual of Police Technique* in which he coined his 'theory of interchange' at the scene (Locard, 1923, 1928, 1930), which in essence states: 'that the person or persons at the scene when a crime is committed will almost always leave something and take something away'.

This doctrine of exchange or transfer is thus based on the observations that:

1. The perpetrator will take away traces of the victim and the scene.
2. The victim will retain traces of the perpetrator and may leave traces of himself on the perpetrator.
3. The perpetrator will leave behind traces of himself at the scene (Wagner, 1986).

It is the principal task of the scientist and scene of crime officer to find, and properly collect and preserve any traces left behind, such as fingerprints, blood stains, fibres from clothing, dirt from shoes, etc., and to locate matching materials on a suspect in order to provide objective evidence that they were present at the scene. This can only be carried out by instituting a systematic search, which will vary in its pattern, depending on the circumstances and type of scene. A number of texts, such as Fisher (1993), recommend several typical search patterns, depending on the type of environment (Figure 4.1). The goal, whatever pattern of search is adopted, is to ensure that all the area in question is thoroughly examined in order to find, document and retrieve all relevant information.

Care must be taken in how the body is handled and moved from its site of initial discovery, as moving the body can lose or confuse evidence – particles fall off, blood swilling washes off materials, etc. In sexual assault murders, moving the body can redistribute body fluids, which can lead to erroneous conclusions. For example, semen can trickle into the anal passage of a victim and give the impression of buggery.

When the body is not present, it can be difficult to interpret blood distribution

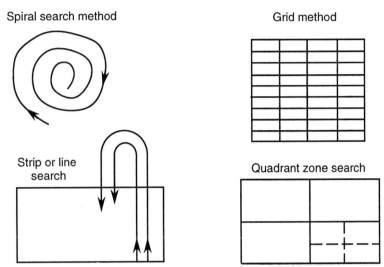

Figure 4.1 Typical systematic search patterns that may be used. The one adopted will depend on the circumstances of the case and type of environment.

patterns, or assess particles from under or alongside the body. Therefore, it is always better for the 'team' to attend when the body is *in situ*. Discussion between the various team members will then allow decisions to be made on the order of examination. It is essential to remember that examining the body means entering, and disturbing the scene.

Examination of the body and the clothing involves the identification of traces or marks, which may have:

- Come from an object. Examples of these may include smears of paint or particles of glass left by a car involved in a fatal hit-and-run accident.
- Been transferred to an object. By Locard's principle there is always the equal likelihood that traces or marks may be transferred to the offending object. As examples, blood, hair, fibres and fabric marks could be transferred from the body to the car.
- Come from the person who carried out the attack. Examples of these are blood stains, semen in rape cases, shoeprints found on the body or on the clothing, and fibres transferred from the assailant's clothing. Particular attention should be directed to sites of attack and defence, e.g., fingernails, hands, forearms and face.
- Come from another scene. Examples of these may be paint fragments or fibres retained on the body, which relate to a different venue from that where the body is found. Finding these may show that a murder occurred elsewhere and the body was dumped in the position where it was found.

We can separate the types of evidence on the body or clothing into: trace evidence, marks on the body and marks in the body.

Trace evidence

These can either be liquids, stains or particulates. The latter are often very small and can be difficult to see on the body *in situ*. It is worth remembering that the forensic scientist can analyse samples that are hardly visible with the naked eye and a great variety of trace material can provide evidence.

Biological traces

These include blood, semen, saliva, nasal and vaginal secretions, fingernails and hairs. Additionally found and sometimes ignored, are fibres and botanical samples. Notes on the collection, packaging and preservation of biological samples are given in the Appendices.

BOTANICAL SAMPLES

These can be useful in locating an outdoor scene of crime, particularly if the body has been moved. They are also useful as an aid in tracing a suspect if there is likely to be any botanical material of a particular type. If the body has been undisturbed for some time, it may also be possible to use botanical evidence either on the body or at the scene to estimate the period of time, either by lack of vegetation under the body or by the amount of growth of plants through bones.

In a case seen by one of us and described in more detail in Chapter 6, roots from a nearby lime tree growing through interred skeletal remains as well as other adventitious growth enabled length of burial to be assessed. The rings of the roots of the tree were especially useful in enabling the botanist to pinpoint within a season, when the deceased had been buried.

CASE 4.1
A further example of the value of such evidence is the finding of a leaf from a potentilla plant inside the pants of a murdered girl found in a garden, although there was no such plant in the vicinity of the body. The sexual assault, which took place before the murder, was in a different location in the garden, and the murderer allowed his victim to get dressed and start to leave before he killed her.

CASE 4.2
Similarly, an abduction of a child occurred and the victim was found under a flowering chestnut tree, which was covered in pollen as was the clothing of the suspect. The latter denied the offence but the pollen level in the clothing was so high it proved the case.

Botanical samples must be retrieved prior to the movement of the body, packaged and transported to the laboratory rapidly, so as not to allow deterioration. In addition, samples of other surrounding vegetation must be taken as controls. In such cases, it is often wise to ensure that a forensic biologist attends the scene. Lichen and mosses, and their disturbance can be useful in cases where it is not known whether someone has jumped from a building or been pushed.

FIBRES AND HAIRS

Fibres and hairs can be found on the body, both on clothing and on skin. Although they may be easily visible, in practice they are usually very difficult to see. It is important to remove these traces before the body is moved and it is also important to ensure that there is no contamination from people present, i.e., as few people as possible should approach the body and they should wear protective clothing. Naked or semi-naked bodies can be taped at the scene. This involves the application of adhesive tape to the body to enable small particles, such as fibres, to be lifted and preserved for examination. However, this should be considered carefully as this could compromise other types of evidence (e.g., fingerprints, paint, etc.). Visible hairs and fibres should be removed at the scene with a pair of untoothed forceps only after they have been photographed *in situ*. Most hairs found in the hands of victims of battery assault and murder are in tufts, and are the victim's own. Sometimes conglomerations of hairs found in the hands of such victims with no obvious orientation of roots at one end may well in fact be related to debris, dirt, etc., lying in the vicinity of the victim, e.g., on the ground where the offence took place. However, fibres from suspects' clothing have been found trapped in fingernails.

BODY FLUIDS

In examining the body prior to removal for post-mortem examination, it is important to note whether any body fluids present could be lost or contaminated during transport. This is particularly important when matching these to the body fluids of the murderer. Thus it is common for swabs to be taken prior to the removal of the body, from the vagina, anus and mouth in murders in which a sexual motive may be present, for the detection of semen. If it is thought that blood from the murderer is present on the body, this should be sampled at the scene, particularly in those cases where movement of the body will result in loss of blood from wounds on the victim contaminating the blood staining present.

CASE 4.3
During a stabbing, the murderer was also cut and blood dripped onto the body of the victim. This was fortunately sampled at the scene, as once the body was moved, blood from the victim's wounds contaminated the area in question.

The taking of samples before the body has been disturbed can also apply to saliva from bite marks. It is sensible to leave the taking of such samples until the post-mortem examination, if there is no risk of contamination. Nasal secretions on a handkerchief at a scene proved vital in the case described below, by providing a link via DNA profiling to the suspect.

CASE 4.4
A 22-year-old woman was found beaten and strangled in a London park. Considering the possibility of linked offences, a murder squad was set up to work alongside a team already investigating a series of rapes in the vicinity. A man's handkerchief left at a site a quarter of a mile from the murder scene was found to be stained with blood and saliva, matching that of the victim. A DNA profile was obtained from a stain of nasal mucus on this handkerchief and found to match the suspect, later arrested for an attempted rape in the same locality (Allard, 1992).

A broken fingernail is another body sample that can provide irrefutable evidence linking a body to a scene. Fingernails have distinct striations that can be matched to the victim (Thomas and Baert, 1965).

BLOOD AT THE SCENE

The presence and distribution of blood at a scene is often central to the investigation. A specialist forensic scientist attending a scene will quite often require further photographs to be taken to show the distribution of blood. In blunt force trauma, the pattern of the blood distribution can be very important and it is possible to measure the angles of blood splashes and spots, and identify sites of attack from these.

DETECTION OF AND IDENTIFICATION OF STAINS AS BLOOD

In most cases where there is a substantial amount of blood present, the need to identify it as such, will not be an issue. In situations where there are only a few stains, or the appearance suggests that the staining is old, then these areas should be screened to ascertain whether or not they are in fact blood. Presumptive tests for blood are based on:

1. The presence of a 'peroxidase'-like enzyme in red blood cells, which catalyses the reduction of hydrogen peroxide and turns phenolphthalein pink (Kastle–Meyer test).
2. Specific reactions for haemoglobin (Takayama test).

Finding blood at a scene requires a systematic approach. Sometimes food and drink stains can be mistaken for blood/body fluids. In addition, the conditions prevailing at the time may make blood stains appear older, owing to heat or humidity, for example. Cleaning up must be considered, particularly when the blood distribution is inconsistent; it can be found by close visual and microscopical examination as well as by chemical detection.

POOLED OR LARGE AREAS OF BLOOD

The appearance of blood, which is in sizeable quantities rather than discrete stains, needs to be assessed in relation to the position of the body and, in particular, in relation to any wounds that are present. The pattern of distribution of such blood stains may indicate whether they were produced during life or after death. Because of the continued ability of blood to clot after death, often one may see areas of clotted blood intermixed with fluid blood. The presence therefore of blood clots at the scene does not indicate that it was shed during life. After death, there is continued oozing of blood from wounds, particularly from those of the head; this may produce substantial areas of blood staining. Care needs to be taken to assess the distribution and quantity of blood with regard to whether or not movement of the body, for resuscitation, for example, has taken place prior to carrying out scene examination. Such movement may cause large quantities of blood to flow from major wounds, such as stab wounds. The blood in these cases originates from collections within the body cavity and, particularly with chest wounds, large quantities may spill out onto the floor on turning the body over.

EVALUATION OF BLOOD DISTRIBUTION PATTERN AT THE SCENE

Blood stains can originate from a number of sources (Figures 4.2–4.9):

1. Sprays produced by impacts to wounds already bleeding.
2. From arterial spurts.
3. Dripping from a blood-filled area.
4. Transference by a weapon (cast off droplets).
5. Smearing from a blood-stained area.
6. Back spatter (typically from the use of firearms).
7. Direct transfer from one object to another, e.g., shoe to floor.

Examination of blood-stain patterns at a scene gives an insight into the actions and activities of victim and assailant, and may be of particular value in assessing the direction of travel of blood spots (by plotting their distribution and angle deposited), their velocity on impact at a surface, e.g., medium velocity of hammer and high velocity of firearm and the distance travelled (MacDonell, 1982). Caution, however, needs to be exercised in the interpretation of blood-stain trajectories and patterns (Pizzola et al., 1986a, b). Stephens and Allen (1983), and Pex and Vaughan (1987) discussed the interpretation of back spatter from firearms, and the latter authors confirmed that such a distribution only occurred with contact or near-contact range wounds unless the surface was already bloody. Forensic scientists, experienced in blood distribution patterns, will use their experience, together with experimental testing and published work, to interpret

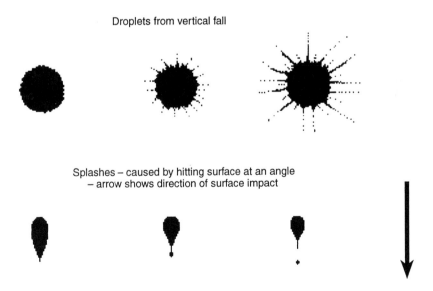

Figure 4.2 Types of blood spots commonly encountered at a scene. The droplets are caused by blood falling vertically. Depending on the distance of the fall and the recipient surface, they may have scalloped edges at shorter distances, or have a more spread out, spiky appearance, with a longer fall. The splashes caused by striking a surface at an angle, have a pear or tear-drop shape. The broader end is where the blood first struck the surface and the tail end indicates where the spot finishes.

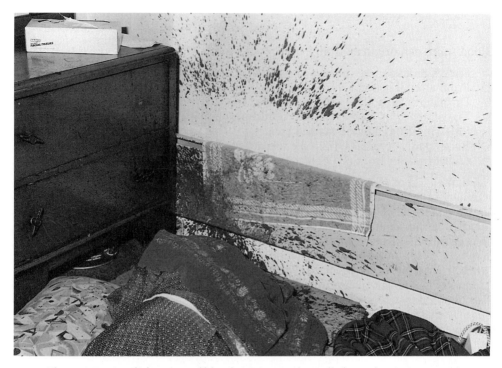

Figure 4.3   A radial pattern of blood staining on the wall above the victim caused
by a blunt weapon repeatedly striking a blood-soaked area of the head
(see also Figure 1.1).

different patterns in order to estimate site of attack and number of impacts. The size and orientation of stains, from spots to splashes, is indicative of the type and location of the attack.

Chemical traces

PAINT

Paint, which may be found on the body or on the clothing of the deceased, can be from wet paint or as a consequence of transference of particles from a painted object. Both smears and spots can originate from wet paint samples and they may be very thin and difficult to see *in situ*. To search for them on the body, it is necessary to use a strong light source and possibly also a single hand lens or magnifier. Particles of paint usually originate from a painted object where the surface coating has chipped off. Such an object may be painted by a single layer of paint or it may have been painted over a period of time by many different layers giving rise to a multilayer paint flake. These paint flakes may be very small and, indeed, the forensic scientist is frequently working with paint flakes smaller than 1 mm in diameter. Larger flakes, which may be seen on the body or clothing, should be removed by tweezers,

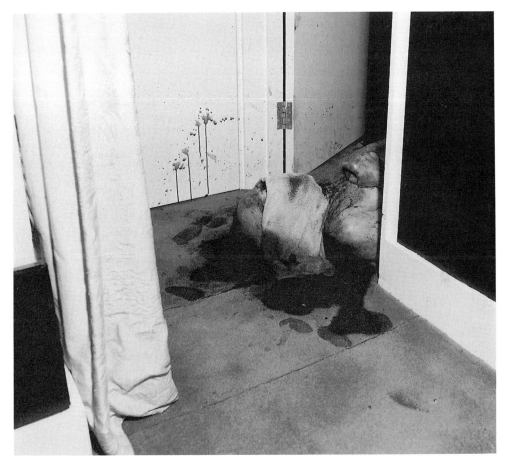

Figure 4.4 Arterial blood spurts on a door near the left side of the deceased's neck. The bleeding had come from the left carotid artery after the neck had been slashed.

providing the lighting is good. If a cluster of very small flakes is seen in a particular location, it can be brushed from the surface and packaged. Although it is possible to retrieve paint flakes on adhesive tape, this is not a recomended method as the adhesive can interfere with any resin analysis, which will subsequently be carried out by the forensic chemist.

Unless paint traces are embedded in the soft tissues of the body, they tend to fall off when the body is moved and it is therefore very important to examine the exposed parts of the body at the scene of death so that particles can be retrieved at this stage.

Paint flakes transferred to clothing are more likely to be embedded in the fibres of the fabric. This can make them much more difficult to find when examining the body *in situ* but they may well not be lost when the body is moved. The clothing sent to the forensic laboratory will have paint particles recovered from it by brushing. To assess the relevance of these particles in the context of the case, it is often useful for the forensic scientist to see the photographs of the clothing on the body *in situ*.

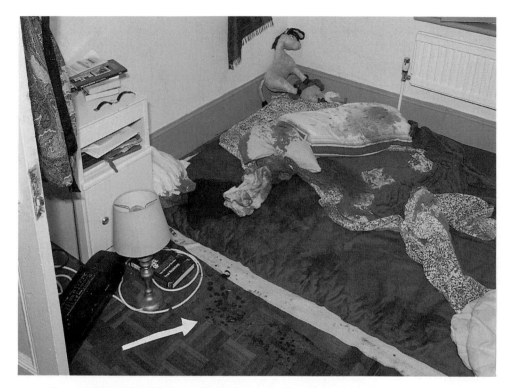

Figure 4.5(a)   Blood that has dripped onto the floor in two clusters near each other. Further heavy blood staining is seen on the nearby bed clothes.

GLASS

Small particles of glass may become embedded in the soft tissues on the surface of the body or transferred to clothing, and may be found in pockets, folds (e.g., trouser turn-ups), socks, shoes and creases in clothing, or scattered in between the fibres of the fabric of the clothing. Glass fragments could originate from a variety of sources, e.g., window, bottle, car windows, ornaments or tableware. The fragments could originate from a clear-glass source or from a coloured one.

The glass fragments may have the typical small 'cube' appearance of toughened glass or they may be thin surface slivers like those obtained from a laminated window. Glass particles can be retrieved in the same way as paint fragments.

Any fragments embedded in the hair, e.g., as a result of an attack with a bottle can be retrieved by combing the hair with a comb seeded by cotton wool or a cellulose fabric such as 'Litex'. A collecting sheet should be held under the head so the particles dislodged fall onto it and can be packaged. If there is a head wound, which is bleeding, it may be necessary to carry out the combing at the scene and before the body is moved. Samples of glass should be collected from the scene for comparison by the laboratory.

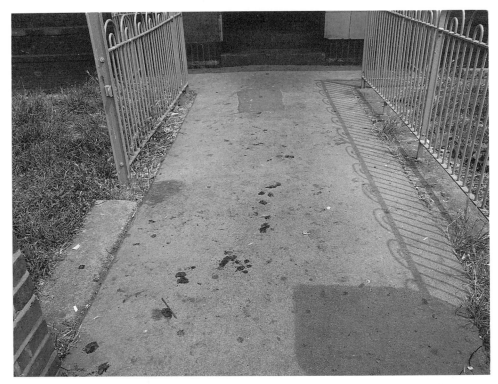

Figure 4.5(b)   Blood that has dripped onto the ground whilst the victim was walking after receiving injuries. Note that the trail is seen from the door (at the top of the picture) from where he had emerged.

PLASTIC

Plastics are made for a variety of purposes and there are many different forms in the environment. Evidential material can range from tiny fragments of polyethylene torn from a plastic carrier bag or rubbish sack, to smears of plastic car bumper material. If they are in the form of particles, they can be picked off the body or clothing. As smears they will normally adhere well to the surface and will not be disturbed when the body is moved. Smears on the body may then be seen and removed during the post-mortem, while smears on the clothing will be found and removed during a subsequent laboratory examination.

SOIL

A deposit of soil on the body or clothing can provide good linking evidence to a particular site. For example, it may be possible to match the soil with a different location from that in which the body is discovered. This can provide evidence of the movement of the person either before or after they were killed.

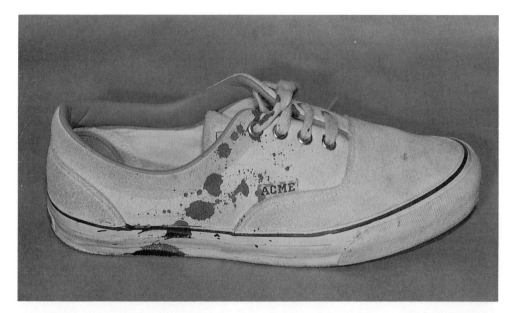

Figure 4.5(c) A blood-stained trainer from the same case as Figure 4.5(b), showing drops on the top of this right trainer.

A significant amount of soil would be needed to enable this to be done satisfactorily; a few particles of quartz are not sufficient.

It must also be emphasised that a forensic geologist is usually required to carry out the comparison of soils and that there are not too many specialists in this field. When undertaking such a task it is necessary to have a full knowledge of the different types of soil in the vicinity of the body. This may require consulting or constructing a comprehensive data bank.

OTHER PARTICULATE MATERIALS

Trace evidence is usually commonly occurring material which is in the 'wrong' place. Therefore, any material could provide potential evidence, as shown in the following example.

CASE 4.6

An attempt was made to glue a woman's nose and mouth with 'superglue' during a long sequence of violent attacks on her which eventually led to her death. Although the body was found in the river, traces of adhesive were still to be seen on her face. Although this finding did not provide *prima-facie* evidence against the suspect, it helped to corroborate the account given by one of the witnesses and thus provided essential evidence at the trial.

Other particulates that have provided evidence, including pieces of ceramic on a body from a household ornament used as a weapon, building materials, such as small

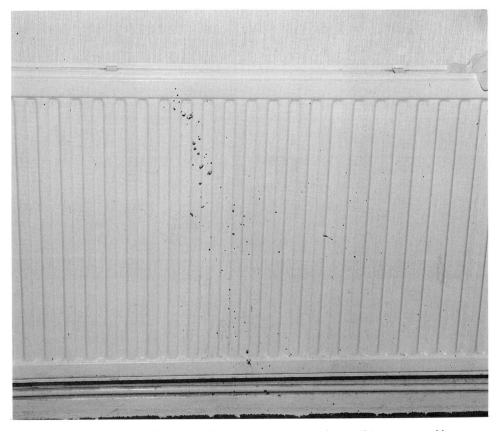

Figure 4.6   A cast-off pattern of blood staining on a radiator. This was caused by blood spraying from the assailant's hammer, which was swung at the head of the deceased as he was attacked whilst on the ground.

fragments of painted plaster or wall cladding, and bundles of fibreglass insulation materials.

STAINS

Stains may result from a variety of materials. In a sexual murder there may be traces of a lubricant on the body or on the clothing of the victim. They need not be removed at the scene provided the examiner is convinced that they will not be disturbed or contaminated when the body is moved. If this is not the case, lubricant on the body should be swabbed off with a clean, dry swab. A control swab should be considered from an adjacent, or preferably contralateral part of the body. If the body is discovered indoors, where it is possible to control and reduce the ambient lighting, it is possible to search for lubricants with an ultraviolet illumination; some lubricants such as Vaseline can fluoresce.

Thick smears of grease are frequently found on the body and clothing of a road

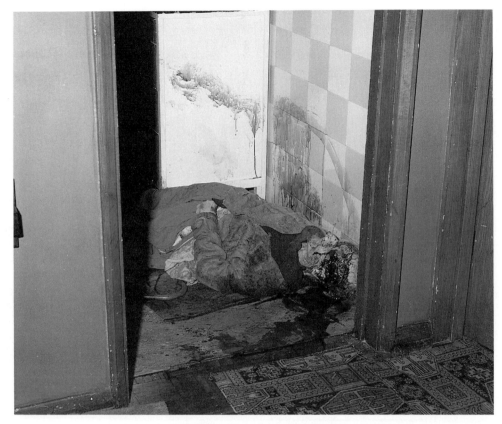

Figure 4.7   Transferred blood from the victim's head and trunk, smeared onto wall in an arc as she fell back onto the floor.

accident. Although it is possible to compare this with the grease from a car, it is often very difficult to interpret the results. One usually hopes that there are some tiny flakes embedded in the grease. Materials like this can be scraped from the body or the clothing with a brand new scalpel blade.

Retrieval of trace evidence

To find these traces, the examiner needs to carry out a thorough visual examination in good lighting conditions. Specialist lighting may be needed, e.g., a laser or ultraviolet source to search for specific materials.

To retrieve traces one can also use:

- Tapings, e.g., for fibres.
- Brushing for particulates, e.g., glass.
- Picking off for particulates, e.g., paint flakes.
- Swabbing for stains, e.g., body fluids.
- Hair combings, e.g., for fibres, gunshot residues.

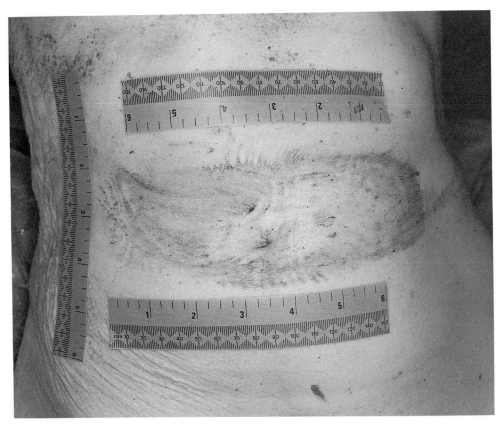

Figure 4.8 A blood-stained shoeprint caused by the deceased being stamped on by the assailant.

Marks on the body

FOOTWEAR IMPRESSIONS

Shoeprints may be on the body itself or on the clothing. On the body they may be in two different forms. They may be in a dust or dirt deposit, which is ingrained on the skin, as a result of a 'stamping'-type transference of materials adherent to the undersurface of the footwear. These marks usually show quite well on the body *in situ*. They should be photographed *in situ*, although it may be necessary to rephotograph a shoeprint at the mortuary after the body has been removed. Specialist lighting conditions give the optimum contrast. Most shoeprints of this type cannot be lifted from the body by an adhesive or gelatin-lifting film. A typical dirty shoeprint is shown in Figure 4.10.

The forceful contact of footwear with the body causes damage to the skin or the underlying tissue, and appears as patterned bruised marks. These marks are usually very stable and can be photographed quite satisfactorily during the post-mortem

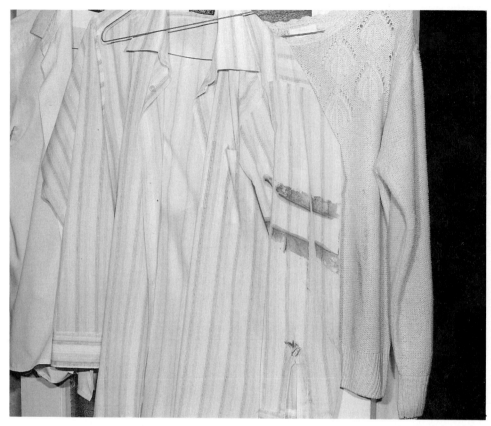

Figure 4.9   Blood staining on a shirt caused by wiping the blade of a knife used in a stabbing.

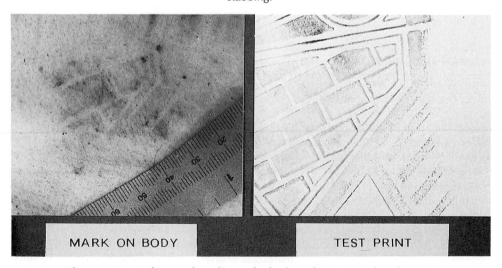

MARK ON BODY   TEST PRINT

Figure 4.10   A shoe mark in dirt on the body and test print taken from it.

examination. Many shoeprint bruises on the face of a victim resulting from kicking or stamping (Figure 4.11) are often accompanied by considerable damage to the soft and bony tissues.

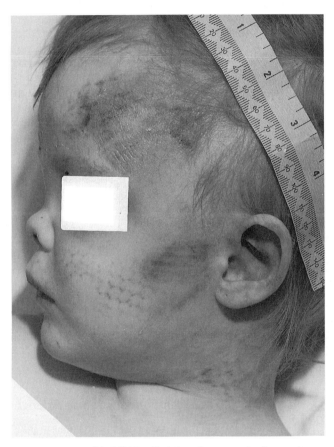

Figure 4.11 A two-year-old child fatally injured as a result of stamping on the head. The trainer shoes of the assailant have produced characteristic patterned bruises. There were severe underlying skull fractures.

The pattern in the footwear imprints can be distorted by the force of the action and it may not be immediately obvious that a particular mark is a shoeprint. Any such mark should be photographed with a scale.

Footwear imprints on the clothing of a victim can be made in a variety of materials, but are commonly in dirt or blood. It can be very difficult to see a shoeprint on a garment when it is examined at the scene, particularly outdoors where it may be difficult to control the level of lighting. At an indoor scene, specialist lighting can be used: a high-intensity white-light source or a fibre-optics source providing ultraviolet wavelengths, or a portable laser giving high-intensity monochromatic illumination are useful methods of illumination (which can cause fluorescence of the shoeprint substrate or of the background fabric). It is clearly easier to find shoeprints on garments after they have been removed from the body and are examined in controlled laboratory conditions. It is therefore important to appreciate that there may be shoeprints on the clothing of a victim at a scene, which may be virtually invisible, so all efforts should be made to preserve them.

For example, shoeprints were found on the inside of a murdered female victim's tee-shirt. The force of the kicks had been sufficient to transfer substances from the surface of the body to the fabric of the shirt, which could then be developed by a variety of staining techniques. If the blood-stained body had been moved before the shirt was cut off, these marks could have been lost, if blood had coated these marks (Hamer and Price, 1993).

Any shoeprint on clothing can be distorted by the folding and creasing of the fabric. It is very useful for subsequent comparison with a pair of shoes, if the scene examiner makes detailed notes and arranges for photographs to be taken of the position of the body and the clothing.

Tyre marks can be found in a similar way on the inside surfaces of clothing of victims of vehicular accidents who have been run over.

FABRIC MARKS

It is possible for marks from a fabric to be left on the body. Bloodstains on the body or on the clothing may show the characteristic pattern of a fabric worn by the assailant. For example woollen gloves may leave a distinctive pattern.

FINGERPRINTS

Fingerprints can be found in a great variety of materials and deposited on the body or clothing. The work of the Serious Crime Unit in the detection of latent fingerprints at scenes is described below.

Serious Crime Unit of the Metropolitan Police Forensic Science Laboratory (London)

The Serious Crime Unit (SCU) was formed in the early part of the 1980s. The team consists of experienced forensic scientists, scientific photographers and fingerprint experts who are given the task of dealing with targeted exhibits from major crime scenes. The success of the work carried out by the unit, which began with the introduction of an argon-ion laser in 1981 (Creer, 1982) for the detection of fingerprints, led to an increased demand for its services at scenes and, in 1985, a transportable frequency-doubled neodymium-yag laser was introduced (Pounds et al., 1986).

Scene examination by the SCU is carried out after the scene has been vetted by an experienced fingerprint officer or scene of crime officer. The scene as far as possible is protected and a full examination is first carried out using a portable Omnichrome laser and Polilight filtered light source. Both these sources have been successfully used to detect evidence left where contaminants are not visible to the naked eye. Any marks or other evidence found is referred to the relevant forensic scientist, fingerprint officer or pathologist, and is then photographed or preserved. Blood pattern analysis by the biologist can be of particular value at this stage to indicate areas of interest. Chemical and physical methods are then carried out by the SCU scientist to enhance shoeprints, fingermarks or other evidence detected during the light examination. Marks in blood where appropriate are sampled for DNA typing and then enhanced with peroxidase reagents, such as leucomalachite green (LMG) or diaminobenzidine (DAB), or a protein stain such as amido black. This is followed by a full fingerprint examination using light and powder. Walls and other surfaces are then treated with iodine followed by ninhydrin to develop latent marks.

Attempts to carry out cyanoacrylate (CNA) fuming at scenes have not proved successful due to the relatively low average humidity in the United Kingdom. Transportable objects are taken back to the laboratory where a full range of sequential techniques are carried out to develop latent fingerprints.

The following two case examples, courtesy of K.E. Creer (personal communication), are typical of the casework of the SCU.

CASE 4.7

An 11-year-old girl disappeared after leaving school and was found 24 hours later in a black polythene sack hidden in a rubbish skip in the corner of the school playground. The skip had been searched previously, so the murderer must have dumped the body after the search commenced. The school caretaker was a strong suspect because he was the last person seen talking to the child but he completely denied any involvement. The SCU was called in the early evening after the body was found and joined the pathologist, fingerprint expert and investigating officers at the scene. The girl's body was still in the sack in the rubbish skip, only the top layer of rubbish having been disturbed to reveal the body. The caretaker's house and his room in the school had been sealed prior to a full examination. The timing was ideal for a laser and ultraviolet examination because it was getting dark by the time the team was assembled at the scene. After a conference it was decided to remove the child's body from the skip and examine it on a body sheet in the school playground rather than risk losing evidence by removing the body straight to the mortuary for the post-mortem examination.

Laser examination of the body using a frequency-doubled neodymium-yag laser revealed a number of fluorescing orange fibres around the child's mouth which were not visible under normal lighting. These fibres were later matched to carpet fibres in an upstairs bedroom in the caretaker's house, and a stain found on this carpet was identified as saliva and was shown to have the same blood group as that of the victim. A partial fingerprint fluoresced on the child's neck and, although, unfortunately, it lacked sufficient detail for identification purposes, it enabled the pathologist to determine that death had been caused by manual strangulation. The soles of the victim's shoes appeared normal until examined under ultraviolet radiation when a light-blue fluorescing powder was visible. This powder was identified as as blue poster-paint powder and matched powder from the floor of the caretaker's room in the school. A fluorescing yellow stain on the child's leg was also sampled. It was not identified but could have provided evidence of where the body had been stored.

Whilst this examination was taking place, the black sack, which had contained the child's body, was being treated in the laboratory and fingermarks later identified as being identical to those of the caretaker were found on the bag using both metal-deposition treatment and cyanoacrylate fuming with rhodamine 6 g staining under laser radiation. The caretaker's house was examined and, as well as finding the stain on the carpet and matching fibres, a complete finger and palm mark was developed by iodine on the wallpaper in the hall. This mark was later identified as being identical with the finger and palm prints taken from the victim.

CASE 4.8

The police were called by a distraught teenage girl early one Sunday morning. Her grandmother with whom she had been staying had been strangled and the girl had been raped by a man who had broken into their home. The SCU were called to the scene, which had been well preserved. The intruder had climbed over a wire fence from an adjoining garden, leaving it bent over. He had attempted to gain access to the premises by breaking a fan vent in the kitchen but had then probably entered through an insecure patio door. Examination of the garden revealed a partly eaten pear lying on the ground by the damaged fence. This pear had obviously been eaten recently as it had not started to deteriorate. The pear was preserved in an exhibits jar in a neighbour's refrigerator, whilst an odontologist was contacted. The scene was then fully examined by laser and ultraviolet radiation. Very few shoe- or fingerprints were found. However, there were stains fluorescing on the carpet in the girl's bedroom so this was preserved for examination. Arrangements were made to meet the odontologist in the laboratory where a number of photographs were taken of the bite marks in the pear. These marks were then cast in silicone rubber. The cooperation between the odontologist and photographer were essential in order to obtain the best possible detail before the pear deteriorated.

Castings taken from a suspect matched the mouldings of the bite marks in the pear. As the pear was still fresh when found, the odontologist was able to draw the conclusion that the teeth marks in the pear were made by the suspect, thus placing him in the rear garden. The stains found on the carpet were identified as semen and gave a DNA profile, which matched that of the suspect.

WOUNDS AND TOOL MARKS

If there is a wound on the body, frequently there is the potential to compare its physical shape and detail with a weapon. Wounds must therefore be preserved from further damage when the body is moved. It should be photographed *in situ* so the scientist can make an assessment of how it might have been made. Bite marks may only be visible on skin in ultraviolet illumination. Although this part of the documentation can be carried out at the post-mortem examination, modern video systems give the potential for viewing the body 'live' when it is illuminated by different wavelengths of light. This, however, may not be possible at the scene, where it is difficult to control the lighting.

Other situations

BODIES WITH LIGATURES OR BINDINGS

In some suspicious deaths, there may be bindings on the body. These can be either self-applied or produced by another person. Bindings, although frequent in auto-erotic deaths, where the person has been unable to free himself, are also to be seen in certain types of sexually related homicides.

The type of knots found can be useful in deciding whether ligatures were tied by the person himself or by another; if they are specialised knots, they may indicate the occupation or experience of the person tying them (Budworth, 1982). It is essential that, where the body can only be moved by removing the binding, then they should be cut at some distance from the knots and the adjoining cuts labelled in such a way that they can be matched again later and the ligatures reconstructed (Figure 4.12).

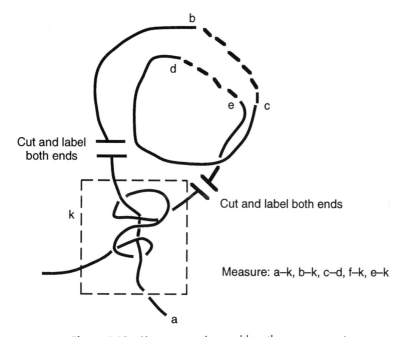

Figure 4.12 Knot annotation and length measurement.

CIRCUMSTANCES INVOLVING ALLEGATIONS OF SUSPICIOUS DEATH WHERE THE BODY IS NOT FOUND FOR SOME TIME OR NEVER FOUND

Such cases, as described below, frequently necessitate the examination of multiple scenes or items.

CASE 4.9
A young child was reported missing and, after quite some time, a bundle of clothing was found in Epping Forest. It was important not only to ascertain whether the clothing belonged to the missing girl but also to see whether there was anything on the clothing that indicated what may have happened to her. It was possible to examine the clothing and, from staining present, state that there was blood shed whilst the garment was being worn. Eventually the body was found buried fairly near to where the clothes were.

CASE 4.10
In a contract killing, no bodies were ever found. However, several scenes were examined to locate possible sites of killing and dismemberment of bodies. Although exhaustive efforts were made by the killers to clear up any evidence, blood staining was

found soaked into floor boards under linoleum and adjoining skirting boards. In addition the remains of zipper teeth were found in a fireplace used to burn evidence. It was possible by grouping the blood found to show that it had originated from more than one person.

BODIES FOUND AT SCENES IN DIFFERENT SITUATIONS FROM WHERE THEY ACTUALLY DIED OR AT AN ENTIRELY DIFFERENT LOCATION

Bodies may be left at scenes by their killers in different situations from where they actually died, so it is particularly important to examine scenes in relation to the body and the actual injuries, ensuring that they are consistent each with the other. Ritualistic murders often leave their victim in certain precise stances, which can thus be useful in identifying serial murders.

Sometimes bodies are buried under piles of bedding or clothes, and furniture is moved around to hide any blood spattering. Attempts are sometimes also made to wash blood staining at scenes. Specialist lighting in such cases is particularly useful.

Ultimately, killers may move victims away from the site of the murder to an entirely different location and also attempt to clear the site of the attack.

CASE 4.11
Two women were found dead in a car in positions where they were obviously not murdered. A cursory look at their flat revealed nothing untoward. However, on closer examination, washed blood staining was found in the hallway and the front steps, indicating that they had been moved after death. The condition of the blood, both in the flat and a small amount on the outside of the car was also useful in indicating the chain of events.

References

Allard J.E. (1992) Murder in South London: a novel use of DNA profiling. *J. For. Sci. Soc.* **32**, 49–58.

Budworth G. (1982) Identification of knots. *J. For. Sci. Soc.* **22**, 327–331.

Creer K.E. (1982) Some applications of an argon ion laser in forensic science. *For. Sci. Int.* **20**, 179–190.

Creer K.E. (1987) The detection and photography of fluorescent marks. *Proceedings of SPIE, The International Society of Optical Engineers*, 743, Fluorescence detection SPIE, pp. 175–179.

Creer K.E. Personal communication.

Fisher B.A.J. (1993) *Techniques of Crime Scene Investigation* 5th edn. CRC Press, Boca Raton, FL.

Hamer P. and Price C. (1993) Case report: a transfer from skin to clothing by kicking – the detection and enhancement of shoeprints. *J. For. Sci. Soc.* **33**, 169–172.

Locard E. (1923) *Manual of Police Technique*. Lyon.

Locard E. (1928) Dust and its analysis: an aid to criminal investigation. *Police J.* **1**, 177–192.

Locard E. (1930) The analysis of dust traces, Part III. *Am. J. Police Sci.* **1**, 496–514.

MacDonell H.L. (1982) *Bloodstain Pattern Interpretation*. Laboratory of Forensic Science, Corning, NY.

Pex J.O. and Vaughan C.H. (1987) Observations of high velocity blood spatter on adjacent objects. *J. For. Sci.* **32**, 1587–1594.

Pizzola P.A., Roth S. and De Forest P.R. (1986a) Blood droplet dynamics – I. *J. For. Sci.* **31**, 36–49.

Pizzola P.A., Roth S. and De Forest P.R. (1986b) Blood droplet dynamics – II. *J. For. Sci.* **31**, 50–64.

Pounds C.A., Creer K.E., Pearson E.F. and Lucas I.T. (1986) *The Use of Non-routine Techniques to Reveal Fingerprints at Scenes of Crime.* A joint Home Office/Metropolitan Police project. Central Research Establishment report no. 600.

Stephens B.G. and Allen T.B. (1983) Back spatter of blood from gunshot wounds – observations and experimental simulation. *J. For. Sci.* **28**, 437–439.

Thomas F. and Baert H. (1965) A new means of identification of the human being: the longitudinal striation of the nails. *Med. Sci. Law* **5**, 39–40.

Wagner G.N. (1986) Crime scene investigation in child-abuse cases. *Am. J. For. Med. Pathol.* **7**, 94–99.

Further reading

Eckert W.G. and James S.H. (1989) *Interpretation of Bloodstain Evidence at Crime Scenes.* Elsevier, New York.

CHAPTER 5

Scene location and associated problems

Attendance at a scene when a decomposed body is found

The discovery of a body after the lapse of a period of days or weeks from the time of death, should always raise the possibility that foul play may be involved. Circumstantial evidence combined with a thorough examination of the site and the body *in situ* will often dispel such anxieties. The pathologist who attends may thus be able to indicate that the cause of death was natural, accidental or suicidal at the earliest possible phase of the investigation, with little further cause for major concern or the deployment of the specialist investigative teams.

When a body or bodies are found out of doors, and/or when there had been attempts at disposal and/or destruction of the remains including by mutliation, suspicions should be raised, and an appropriate and thorough investigation of the scene is essential in all such instances. It would be foolhardy to deny that the examination of a scene where a decomposed body is found, is particularly difficult and unpleasant, and it must be re-iterated from the outset that such investigations are perhaps the most difficult.

The main points to be mindful of in such circumstances are:

1. The general features and sequence in which the changes of decomposition occur, and particularly how artefacts could be produced that may simulate ante-mortem injuries or other signs that would lead one to the opinion that foul play was involved.
2. The collection of all relevant materials and trace evidence, and the cataloguing and documentation of the appropriate observations, which would assist in the reconstruction of the death and the timing of death.
3. The positive identification of the deceased at as early a stage as possible in order that the investigation be directed more appropriately and more specifically to a particular individual, thus enabling valuable and crucial historical and circumstantial evidence to be brought to bear on the investigation.
4. To ascertain the possible cause of death and a possible motive for homicide if it is suspected.

Stills photography and video-recording of scenes is discussed in detail in Chapter 2, although it is worth emphasising that, with outdoor scenes, in some instances aerial photography may be useful in order to pinpoint the exact position of the body and the site of its disposal in relation to nearby roadways and other landmarks.

The available obvious access to the site where the body is found must be carefully inspected. The movement of vehicles to and from the site, and relevant tyre and footwear impressions may be of importance in the eventual reconstruction. Indeed a path, other than the one that is the common and established 'right of way', may need to be designated early on and marked out with tape to ensure that there is as little disturbance of the scene as possible.

Protective clothing must be made available to all those who are directly involved in such an investigation. In addition to the unsuitability of the terrain and the general unpleasantness of the cadaver, various micro-organisms will thrive in great abundance throughout decomposed bodies. These include *Clostridium* species and abundant Gram-negative (particularly coliform organisms) and Gram-positive organisms (including micro-aerophilic or anaerobic Streptococci). Any contamination with, or worse still, any inoculation from needle-stick injuries of such bacteria into those handling or in contact with the body can have very unpleasant and even fatal consequences.

Decomposed bodies are often covered in an occasionally spectacular growth of moulds on exposed surfaces. These belong to *Penicillum*, *Aspergillus* and *Mucor* species, and produce large numbers of spores, particularly if an attempt is made to move the body. Inhalation of these shed spores may lead to respiratory problems, more so in those with an atopic disposition. Protective masks should be worn for this purpose.

In bodies found out of doors, exuberant mushroom growths are often seen in the immediate vicinity of the body and may indeed direct the attention of passers-by to the body.

Any injuries sustained on site during the investigation of such 'scenes', and all other medical complaints, no matter how trivial, must be reported, documented and attended to carefully. Ignac Semmelweiss allegedly contracted septicaemia when handling a decomposed body in the autopsy room in 1865 and died of the same disease that he had tried so hard to eradicate from obstetric wards (Findley, 1948).

The pathologist is often the only medical person on site and should therefore appraise the other members of the investigative team of the various possible health hazards.

The scene

A decomposed body may be found indoors, or more frequently, out of doors, either on the surface, partially or completely buried to varying degrees, or in water.

INDOORS

In the modern, egocentric and less caring society, with the loss of the extended family as a frequently encountered unit, it is increasingly common for elderly persons who are living apart from their families, particularly those who are of a reclusive or introverted personality, to die without their absence being noticed for several days. Only after an interval has elapsed, and largely by accident, is the body discovered by chance visitors, council or other workers, or callers to the house, or by neighbours worried about agitated pets or by the stench of putrefaction.

In such instances it is often found that these deaths are due to natural causes, occasionally suicide, hypothermia or accidental causes (e.g. carbon monoxide poisoning). Sometimes the death is precipitated by a fall with a lower limb fracture, with the deceased being unable to seek or obtain assistance.

It should become apparent early on in the investigation that death has come unexpectedly when the deceased is found in a completely undisturbed bed, or sitting fully clothed in front of a television set, which is turned on, or resting on a sofa. The house is secure and there is no evidence of a disturbance or break in. Unfinished food or drink may be in close vicinity to the deceased and mail is frequently found piled up untouched behind the door or in the letter box. These cases are often dealt with by uniformed police officers (together with the coroner's officer) with the body being only presented to the mortuary for autopsy without a full 'scene of crime' investigation being carried out.

When a body is found indoors it is important to assess the prevailing temperature inside the house prior to windows and doors being opened and left open. In those instances when the central heating has been switched on fully for several days after the death had taken place or when electrical conductor bar heaters are in close proximity to the body, the rate of putrefaction is markedly accelerated, with changes that more usually would have taken a few days to appear in temperate climates, becoming prominent very early on.

In all such cases, it is important to seek a full medical history of the deceased from the local community hospital, health centre, general practitioner and/or community nurse. Such investigations can then be quickly wound up.

Police officers dealing with such cases that appear *prima facie* to be somewhat unusual should be encouraged to obtain a second opinion at an early phase; evidence of unclothing, injury or signs of a disturbance should require an early visit from officers trained in homicide investigation. It is extremely difficult, if not impossible, to attempt to retrieve the situation when a scene has already been variously altered and disturbed from its original state. It is the counsel of perfection to attempt to record all such instances photographically.

When a body inside a house is found to be partially or totally concealed, or in an unusual location within the house such as in an attic, outbuilding, garage or cellar, or perhaps concealed within a wardrobe or underneath floor boards or up a chimney, then the possibility of foul play must be considered at a very early stage, and every effort made to collect carefully and methodically as much evidence as possible to exclude this. The discovery of bodies of infants, children and/or younger adults, particularly in similar circumstances, should always raise strong suspicion. The same is perhaps more obvious when there have been attempts at disposal of the body such as by partial burning, the use of chemicals or acids, or by dismemberment. In all such circumstances a full scene of crime investigation is imperative.

Tissue damage of a very extensive nature can be produced by pets who are locked inside the house with no other access to food (Rossi et al., 1994). Animals will start by licking away at secretions emerging from the body orifices but soon after will eat away at the soft tissues. Access to the body by rodents and by ants may cause further injuries after death, which may be quite confusing to interpret.

OUTDOORS

Bodies will often be discovered out of doors accidentally by members of the public and a decision to treat the case as suspicious should be made at an early stage by the officers who are first on the scene. In those instances when the discovery of the body is the result of an anonymous tip-off to the police, more caution is required from the outset.

The person may have died there or could have been transported to or deposited at such a site from another locus some distance away. In the case of a deceased person found by the seashore, the question arises as to whether the person has died at the site of discovery or has been washed up by the tide from out at sea. The following example posed just such a question.

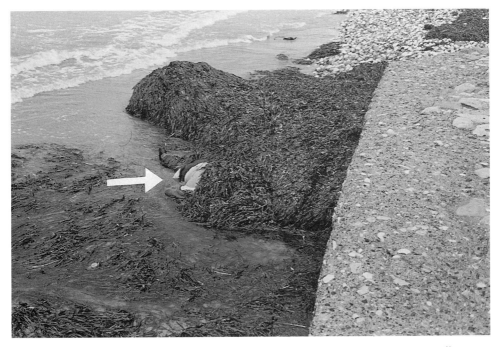

Figure 5.1(a)   A view of the harbour wall and the deceased, who is lying partially hidden by seaweed.

CASE 5.1
A 60-year-old male was found caught up within seaweed by a harbour wall as shown in Figure 5.1(a). The man was initially unidentified and it was not known whether he had entered the water from one of the ships just outside the confines of the harbour or gone in from the harbour wall. The autopsy showed that he had a stab wound to his left upper arm, and an incised wound to the back of his head and to the palm of his right hand. Examination of his left leg and left arm revealed superficial friction marks indicative of contact with the stones from the harbour wall near where he had been found (Figure 5.1(b) and (c)). After enquiries were made locally, it was established that a man, later identified as the deceased, had been involved in a knife

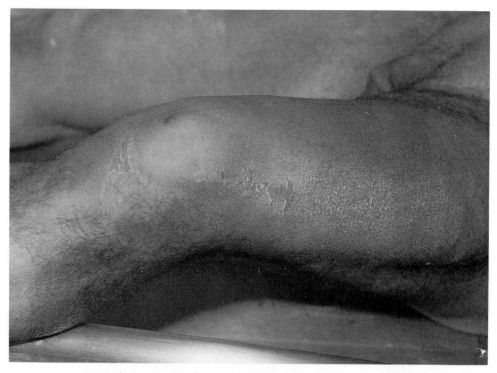

Figure 5.1(b) The left leg showing superficial friction abrasions.

fight with two men. He had apparently lost his balance and fallen over the harbour wall into the water and drowned.

Persons intent on commiting suicide, often try to conceal their deed and secrete themselves in woods or undergrowth, often many miles away from their neighbourhood, to avoid detection or a disturbance of their plans. In such very secluded circumstances, they may take overdoses, hang themselves, or less commonly fatally injure themselves by firearms or cutting implements, well out of the way of the public gaze. Months may elapse before such human remains are discovered.

The mode of death may be quite obvious in such cases from the examination of the scene, in the shape of empty bottles of tablets or syringes close by the body, or as ligatures from which the body is still suspended. If sufficient time has elapsed, ligatures made of organic material may deteriorate by moisture or less sturdy ones may snap, with the body being found on the ground with only the remnants of the ligature around the neck and on the suspension point above the body.

Post-mortem damage including disarticulation could be caused by wild animals (Hill, 1977; Haglund et al., 1988; Bruce and Rao, 1991; Hyams and Rao, 1991; Haglund and Reay, 1993) and these changes would be superimposed on the putrefactive changes thus causing further potential difficulties in interpretation. Bodies may be dismembered and partially unclothed in such circumstances, with different parts of the body being found at vastly separate locations. These changes may resemble those of a terminal struggle.

An early search of the pockets may reveal a suicide note or some other form of

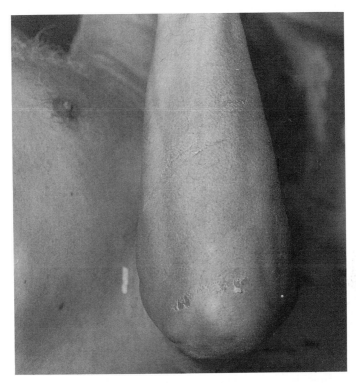

Figure 5.1(c)   The left arm showing superficial friction abrasions.

identification through which the identity of the missing person can be traced, and any predisposing psychiatric background identified at an early stage.

Persons may die from exposure; this is either induced by cold and/or moist weather on its own, or aided by exhaustion or the liberal use of alcohol, and less frequently of other substances. It is important to remember the well-documented association of such deaths from hypothermia with 'paradoxical undressing' (Gormsen, 1972; Wedin et al., 1979; Sivaloganathan, 1986). The body may be partially undressed or totally naked in such instances, and this often raises the possibility of a sexual crime and foul play on initial examination. Certain cases, which at first sight appear to have been death from exposure in hikers or bikers, will turn out to be homicides, often with a robbery or sexual motivation.

In the instance of bodies transported to a site to effect their disposal and to prevent their discovery, it is often the case that there will be an attempt to dispose of, or conceal the body further by covering it with vegetation, burning it or by burying it in a shallow grave. Chemical agents such as acid or quicklime may be added in an attempt to accelerate decomposition. The procedure for the recovery of human remains from clandestine graves is discussed elsewhere in this chapter.

In such instances it should be borne in mind that, if a weapon has brought about the death, it may be left with the body or discarded very close to it. It is therefore important that any search of the scene should not be limited to the site where the body is found but should also be expanded further afield as circumstances dictate. Blood-stained clothing belonging to the assailant may also be disposed of close by. ABO blood grouping may still be carried out satisfactorily on such material (Lee et al., 1988; Kubo, 1989), although nowadays DNA analysis is more commonly employed.

Timing death from decomposition

The estimation of the time of death from features of decomposition that can be observed internally and externally is fraught with inaccuracy in that there are so many potential variables involved, not all of which may be acting simultaneously or in sequence. Individual components cannot be extricated one from another and therefore experimental situations are difficult to control. What may hold true for one particular set of conditions, environment or climate, may differ from another situation.

The information that is available is derived from three main sources (Rodriguez and Bass, 1985; Mann et al., 1990):

1. Observed changes in human cadavers in whom the exact date of death is known but the body is not found till some time afterwards.
2. Observations on non-human material; in particular, studies have been carried out on the putrefaction rates of frozen, thawed, and mechanically injured rats and the carcasses of pigs.
3. The information obtained from controlled studies in human cadavers. The Department of Anthropology of the University of Tennessee examined changes occurring in 150 bodies of adults of both sexes from three ethnic origins. They included homicide victims and bodies donated to medical science or unidentified persons.

VARIABLES FOUND TO HAVE AN EFFECT ON DECAY

Ambient temperature

During cold or freezing weather the decay rate is greatly reduced, or ceases completely. Cold weather does not effect the maggots that already lie inside the body; they will continue to be active within the body cavities because they produce their own heat.

In warm to hot weather an exposed body may become nearly skeletalised within 2–4 weeks. Cold weather may delay or even prevent decay other than skin discoloration and the appearance of mould patches on the surface of the body. At those times of the year when the temperature fluctuates between cold and warm, the rate of decay is very variable and is even more difficult to assess in relation to post-mortem interval.

Humidity

In arid areas, desiccation and mummification may occur at an early phase, and this prevents infestation with insects. Increased humidity, conversely, accelerates the rate of decay and infestation with insects.

Soil pH

This appears to have little direct effect on the rate of decay. Additives to the soil such as quicklime may accelerate putrefaction.

Access to the body by insects

The quicker and more diffuse the access of flies to the body with the laying of their eggs and their maturation to pupae, the faster the rate of decay. This is perhaps the most significant factor in the rate of decomposition. The first flies may land on a body placed in a wooded area within seconds from deposition of the body in warm or hot weather. Any wounding of the body or discharge from any orifice will attract insects.

Dimensions of the body

Although on the basis of logical principles, the rate of decay should be related to the height, weight and build of the body, this is not borne out in experimental studies. Probably the main reason for this is that adipose tissue becomes liquefied at a very early phase by autolytic and bacterial processes, and as such is lost by melting away from the body.

Clothing and other coverings around the body

Clothing serves to protect parts of the body from the direct effects of sunlight; maggots tend to avoid direct sunlight and thus the protected areas decompose more quickly from maggot infestation. This decomposition thus tends to commence where clothing is creased as in crotch, armpits, collar area and natal cleft.

If the body lies within a receptacle such as a body bag or shroud, decomposition is also delayed as there is no access by insects to the body. Madea (1994) reported the case of a dismembered corpse, which was found 2 years after death, wrapped in plastic bags, 30–50 cm deep in loose earth. The whole body, as well as internal organs, were well preserved because of the air-proof conditions in which the remains were found.

Surfaces on which the body is placed

Placing the body on concrete would delay decay but accelerate the features of mummification.

Exposure to the elements

Direct rainfall does not seem to affect the rate of decay, in particular, after the skin has hardened enough to produce a protective covering to the rest of the body.

Activity of rodents and carnivores

Animals will eat away parts of the body, particularly the cancellous bones and the bone ends of the long bones, and also the pelvis. Bones may be carried away after disarticulation up to one and a half miles from the site of deposition of the body. Rats and mice gnaw away at soft tissues, particularly at the extremities, and will tend to burrow into the main body cavities.

The absence of any evidence of rodent or carnivore feeding may suggest that the body was only moved to the exposed area shortly before its discovery.

As a rule of thumb, in temperate climates, within the first 3 days there is a brownish discoloration of the surface veins, softening of the eyeball and some greenish discoloration of the skin of the right iliac fossa. After 3 days, the greenish discoloration extends over all the abdomen and to other parts of the body; there is marked swelling of the external genitalia and brownish green discoloration of the scrotum and vagina. Within the next 3–5 days the abdomen is bloated with gases under pressure and there is eyeball liquefaction. Blisters and bullae form on the skin surface. The nails loosen and fall off at about 2–3 weeks. The hair may also fall off in tufts but tends to lie at the original site where the body was deposited even if the body has been attacked by animals.

Bodies that are found in water as a rule decompose slower than those in air, except if the water is heavily polluted with organic waste.

Adipocere, which results from the saponification of the body fats, has a wax-like consistency, frequently has a light coloration and is usually, although not exclusively, seen in warm, damp and anaerobic conditions (Mant and Furbank, 1957; Simonsen, 1977; Takatori et al., 1986; Cotton et al., 1987). It may be seen within weeks, but more usually, over a period of several months. Experimentally it has been shown to occur in warm water submersion (15–21 °C) from about 2 months (Mellen et al., 1993).

Identification in decomposed bodies

Particularly if foul play is suspected, personal identification of the deceased at an early stage in the investigation is essential.

In the bodies that are found in a secure scene indoors, circumstantial evidence may enable an almost certain identification of the deceased, given that the features of the deceased fit those of the known occupant of the house. Decomposition may alter appearances, in particular the bloating caused by gaseous production may cause a casual untutored observer to assume that the deceased was much more obese than the person was known to be during life, with the possibility of mistaken identity. Many articles, documents as well as the location itself may give excellent pointers to identity and therefore all such information must be documented and preserved where appropriate. It is also useful to photograph the body, particularly when it is taken from one type of environment to another, for example, recovery of a body from a cold river to relatively warm open air. Photography at this stage, with a close up of the face, is often useful, because in many instances by the time the deceased is removed to the mortuary for autopsy, there is a rapid progression of decomposition with consequent deterioration in the facial appearance. Detailed identification from information gained at the scene will be carried out at a later stage either in the mortuary or laboratory and is beyond the scope of this text to discuss methods of identification in further detail.

Investigation of buried and partially concealed remains

The investigation of sites where there is suspicion of concealment of human remains following homicide is a complex operation and will depend on the prevailing circumstances.

Searching for human remains

It is convenient here to consider briefly the general principles involved in searching for a body, and particularly in situations where there is deliberate concealment.

Such a task involves, in many instances, substantial deployment of manpower and equipment. The type of specialists, equipment and vehicles used, will depend on the locality of the search, climatic conditions, type of environment (whether land or water), whether the person has been buried or concealed in some other way, and for how long. In the search for a particular grave, the assistance of aerial photography, including the occasional use of an infrared thermal camera, has a useful part to play (Dickinson, 1977; Killam, 1990). In addition geophysical techniques (Gaffney and Gater, 1993), well established in the field of archaeology, also have clear forensic applications. The use of specially trained dogs in the detection of recently interred remains has on occasions proved particularly useful (Vanezis et al., 1978). A recent project examining the multidisciplinary approach to the investigation of clandestine graves was set up in Colorado (France et al., 1992). The study involved burying six pigs and applying various methodologies to detect the burial sites including aerial photography, geophysics (magnetics, electromagnetics, ground penetrating radar, soil gas, metal detector), geology, botany, entomology, thermal imagery and sniffer dogs.

The health and safety of the search team must not be overlooked. Personnel must be adequately protected, particularly where a search is contemplated in a hazardous location or under adverse conditions.

Types of graves

A grave is essentially a place where human remains are buried. They may contain persons interred in the normal manner following the legally accepted procedure for disposal, or they may be clandestine.

CLANDESTINE GRAVES

Clandestine graves may be categorised from the point of view of forensic investigation, under the following headings.

Mass grave

1. The persons buried may be the victims of war crimes and the site contains human remains which have been buried, usually at the same time.
2. Homicide victims killed by one or more individuals are buried at the same or at different times in the same site.

Multiple grave

One grave that contains a small number of individuals, e.g., all the members of one family.

Grave containing one individual

This is the most common situation encountered by most forensic pathologists.

Recovery of human remains

PARTIALLY BURIED BODY

With a partially concealed body, recovery is carried out in the same way as if the body was fully buried, bearing in mind that it may be in an advanced state of decomposition and care must be taken to recover the remains in a complete state and without causing post-mortem damage.

FULLY BURIED BODY

The procedure for the recovery of a fully buried body is essentially the same, whether from a clandestine grave or as part of the process of exhumation from consecrated ground.

Recovery must be carried out slowly and carefully, paying attention at all times to the need for the collection of all the remains and any consensual artefacts, in an undamaged and complete state. In view of the length of time the task may take, some may find it more comfortable to dig a trench in which to stand, parallel to the burial plot.

In certain cases the advice and active participation of archaeological expertise has proved invaluable (Hunter, 1994) but can never replace active participation and supervision by the forensic pathologist. It is the latter who has the overall responsibility for ascertaining the cause of death, evaluating any injuries and giving guidance on identity, length of internment, etc.

The earth surrounding the body may reveal considerable information and should therefore be dug up systematically. Initially, the soil must be removed from all sides of the burial site and placed in bags which are then labelled with the area of retrieval. One should use a small stainless steel garden trowel in order that soil can be removed with the minimum of disturbance to the underlying skeleton. On occasions, a builder's small pointed trowel can be used when delicate removal is necessary. Cheaper painted items of equipment are known to contaminate scenes.

The soil should then be sieved through a 2 cm ($^3/_4$") mesh. If this is not carried out, one runs the risk of not finding small bones of the hands, wrists, feet, hyoid bone, teeth, in addition to non-human items, such as bullets or jewellery.

The need to take soil samples not only from the area around the body, or coffin, but from other locations in the cemetery for instance, was emphasised by Camps (1962). This is particularly important in excluding any noxious substances, especially arsenic. He described a case where the presence of arsenic in soil samples completely invalidated estimates of the poison within the remains in the coffin.

Once the body has been exposed, the soil is cleaned off it, then plastic sheeting and sometimes hardboard is placed beneath it to aid removal. Contamination of the body, which may interfere with the autopsy should be taken into account.

Removal of the body in a complete state may be difficult, especially if virtually skeletalised. Bones must therefore be collected and placed in separate bags, and labelled for ease of recognition.

Vegetation may prove to be extremely useful for estimating the length of interment. Roots, in particular, which have grown through parts of the body may prove invaluable, as in the following case. The advice of a botanist in such cases should be sought at an early stage and indeed the botanist should attend the site wherever possible.

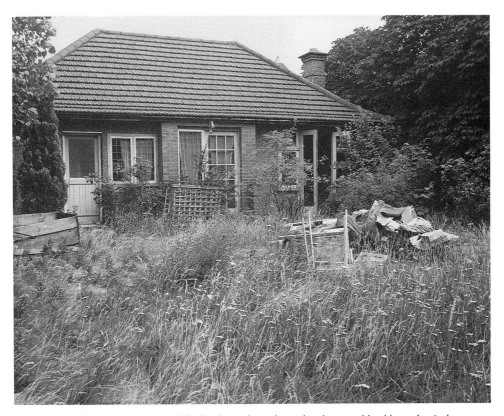

Figure 5.2(a)   A view of the back garden where the deceased had been buried.

CASE 5.2
A fully clothed female skeleton, which had been buried in the back garden of a bungalow, was discovered with the help of specially trained dogs. The deceased had been buried 0.3 metres beneath the surface and adjacent to a mature lime tree hard by a wall. Nearby was a plastic bag with the remains of an adult domestic fowl (*Gallus gallus*). The bird was in a lesser state of decomposition than the human remains because it was contained within a plastic bag. The soil was removed using a stainless steel trowel so that there would be minimum disturbance to the skeletal remains.

When the skeleton had been fully exposed, plastic sheeting was placed beneath the remains and carefully introduced under the entire length of the skeleton to ease it from the site (Figure 5.2(a)–(d)). It was essential to identify the remains, find a cause of death and estimate the length of interment. Identity was achieved by comparing ante-mortem hospital X-rays and clinical notes with the skeletal remains. The deceased had been stabbed and cuts were found in her clothing, and corresponding injuries to her ribs and sternum. The length of burial was estimated from examination of vegetation, which had grown through the skeleton and included adventitious roots from the lime tree. Three methods were used for dating, taking into account root injury, root growth and branch injury. It was estimated that the skeleton had been in the soil for 5 years, which was approximately the time since

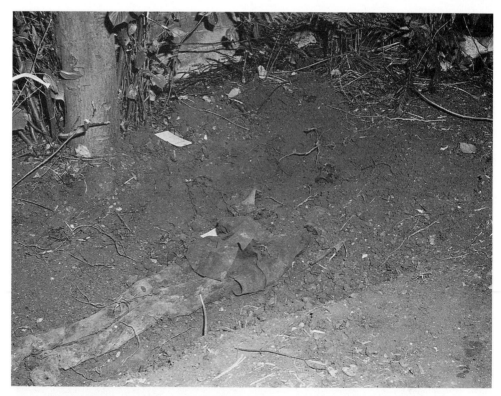

Figure 5.2(b)   A shallow grave beside a lime tree. The remains have been partially uncovered. Note the number of roots from the tree, which have grown within the grave and through clothing.

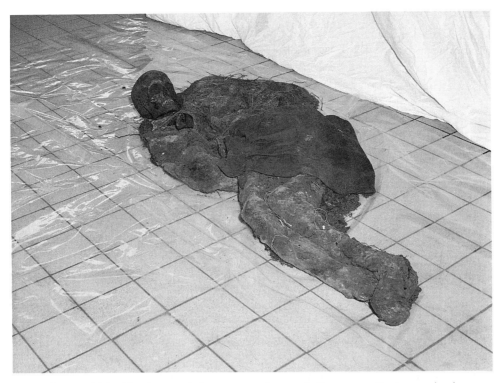

Figure 5.2(c)   The deceased after recovery from a shallow grave. Roots can clearly be seen with the remains.

the victim had last been seen alive. For a fuller account of this case the paper by Vanezis et al. (1978) should be consulted.

The coverings of the body, which must be carefully collected, will often provide invaluable evidence in assisting identification of the body. In addition, they may sometimes (as in the previous case) give invaluable pointers as to the manner of trauma leading to death, particularly if the remains are skeletalised and are incomplete as a result of action by predators, as in the following case.

CASE 5.3
A 14-year-old schoolgirl was abducted and killed by her stepfather. He was convicted and jailed prior to finding her remains. Whilst in prison, he informed the prison authorities that he had placed the body of his stepdaughter within a disused cemetery. Eventually her remains were found incomplete, scattered and partially buried by the overgrowth of vegetation and leaf mould (Figure 5.3(a)–(d)). Her clothing was found and identified by her mother. On her jumper there were two types of damage: tears from animal teeth and linear tears typical of having been caused by a sharp implement such as the blade of a knife. The tears were distributed over the left front of the jumper and on the left sleeve. It appeared therefore that she had been stabbed repeatedly and had tried to defend herself by attempting to fend the knife off with her left arm, thus receiving defensive wounds to this region. Amongst the skeletal remains a section of rib was identified which had a clean cut,

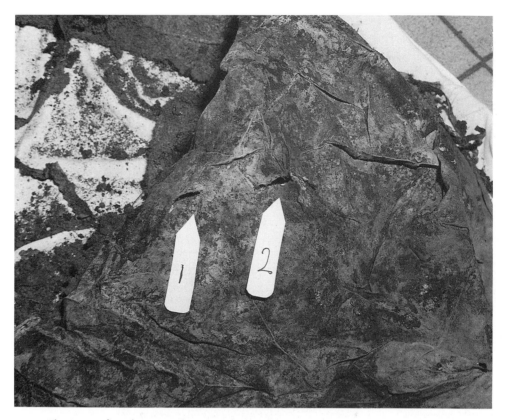

Figure 5.2(d) The internal aspect of a lace blouse showing cuts caused by a knife used to stab the deceased.

confirming the fact that she had received at least one injury to the chest from a sharp implement (Figure 5.3(e)).

Exhumation of legally interred remains

Occasionally, in order to investigate fully a case that has been legally disposed of by burial, it is necessary to exhume the body. A typical situation may concern the burial of a deceased with the usual formalities of disposal adhered to (death having been thought to have been due to some non-suspicious cause), which at a later date, in the light of further information, may indicate that there could be some element of foul play involved.

For the sake of completeness, in addition to the scenario described above involving a criminal investigation, exhumations may also be carried out for:

- Possible civil proceedings.
- Identification.
- Redevelopment of graveyard (most common).
- For ancient or historical reasons.

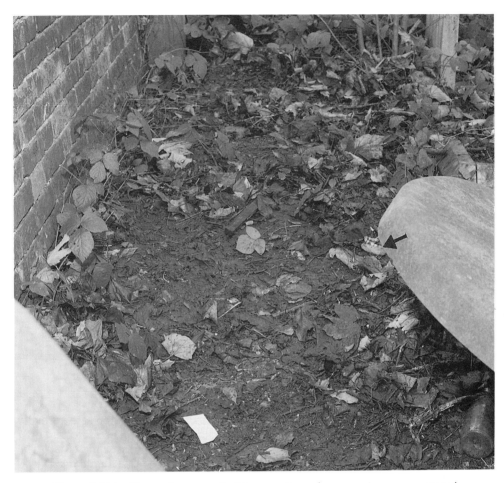

Figure 5.3(a) The perimeter wall of the cemetery where remains were scattered.
The mandible of the deceased is just visible (arrowed).

It should be appreciated that the legal procedure for exhumation varies, in some cases significantly, between different countries and jurisdictions, and is not relevant to our discussion here.

As with recoveries from clandestine graves, certain precautions must be observed and procedures adhered as well as fulfilling the legal requirements for disinterment of a body in such circumstances.

The most important aspect of the procedure at the graveside, is to exhume the correct body. Stringent requirements for identification must therefore be adhered to. Positive identification of the grave, wherein lies the deceased in question, is the responsibility of the cemetery authorities. The graveyard superintendent or some other cemetery official must, therefore, be present at the graveside to do this and the official should indicate the actual plot that is to be opened.

As with other outdoor scenes, it is essential to work in an environment that is free of interference from unwanted onlookers. For this reason, and also to avoid the

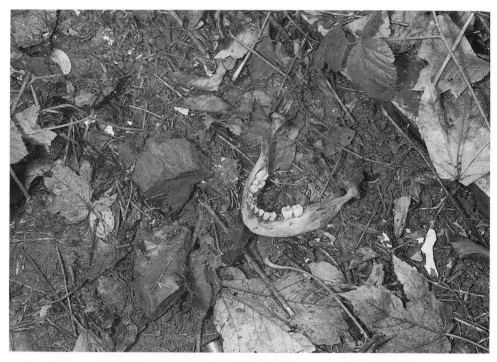

Figure 5.3(b)   A close-up view of the mandible lying amongst vegetation and leaf mould.

procedure interfering with the daily routine of the cemetery, exhumations are normally carried out early in the morning at first light. In addition, the site is also screened off.

Initially, the grave site is dug to a sufficient depth in order to expose the coffin. The coffin plate should then be identified, preferably by the original undertaker who interred the body. At this stage samples of soil may need to be taken from all sides surrounding the coffin and from other parts of the cemetery, if poisoning is suspected (see above).

The coffin is then lifted and should be removed to the mortuary after removal of excessive mud; care must be taken in removal of a coffin which is disintegrating. In common with all scenes, documentation as discussed in Chapter 2 is essential. The gravside aspect of the exhumation is thus completed with the removal of the body from the cemetery to the mortuary for autopsy.

CASE 5.4

Allegations were made that an elderly male in a nursing home had been maltreated. He had apparently been struck on the head, or had been pushed and then struck his head. The exact circumstances of his death were not entirely clear. The deceased died about a week after the incident which at the time had not been alleged. No autopsy was carried out and the deceased was buried in a local cemetery. Eighteen months later when there was general disquiet regarding the treatment of some of the elderly patients in the particular nursing home, it was felt that an exhumation should be carried out in this case as death had occurred soon after the alleged

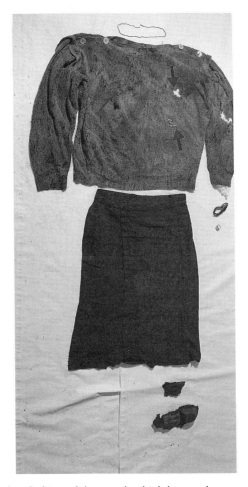

Figure 5.3(c) The clothing of deceased, which her mother was able to identify.
Note tears in the cardigan due to animal teeth (upper arrow) and from stabbing by a
knife (lower arrow).

incident (Figure 5.4(a)–(e)). The autopsy was able to confirm that there was no substantial head injury causing fracture to the skull or any evidence of intracranial staining from blood products as a result of an intracranial haemorrhage. The rest of the organs were still in a remarkably good state of preservation to enable a general gross assessment of trauma to be made but natural disease could not be confirmed with confidence.

Factors affecting decomposition after burial

The condition in which the body is found may be affected by a number of factors following burial. These have been studied by Mant (1953) during the course of war

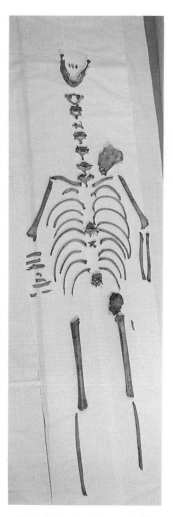

Figure 5.3(d) The human skeletal remains recovered from the cemetery. They were incomplete and comingled with animal bones, from which they were separated.

crimes investigation work, in which he examined a large number of exhumed bodies from Nazi concentration camps in Europe. They include:

1. *The state of the body before death.* A grossly emaciated body at the time of death may decompose into a skeleton very rapidly, whereas a well-nourished body buried at the same time and under the same circumstances shows far less decomposition.
2. *The time elapsed between death and burial, and environment of the body during this period.* Mant observed that when aircrew found at different intervals after death, within a few days of each other, were buried in the same cemetery, those buried first were less decomposed.

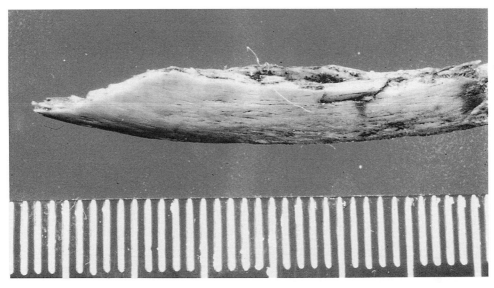

Figure 5.3(e)   A section of rib showing a clean cut edge produced by a knife.

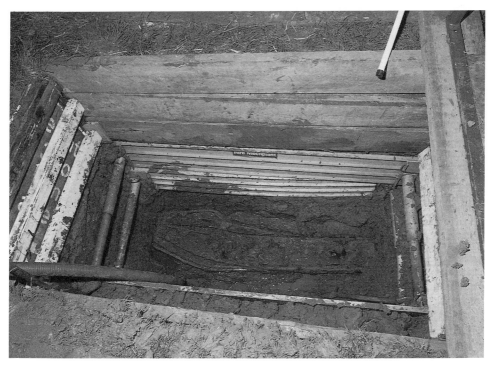

Figure 5.4(a)   A view of the burial plot, which had been dug down to expose the top of the coffin. Note that, particularly in this case where the soil was liable to collapse into the plot, supports were placed on both sides to secure the grave.

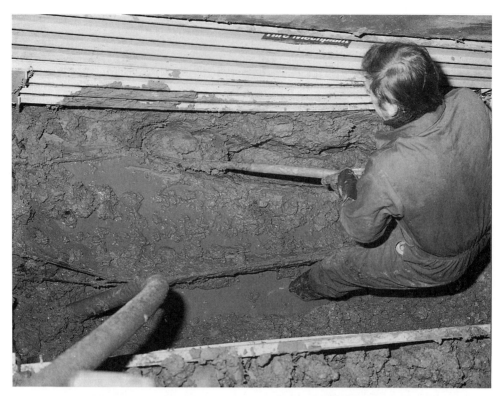

Figure 5.4(b) The soil in this case was clay and had retained a great deal of water, which had to be drained away whilst the soil was being removed from the sides of the coffin.

3. *Effect of a coffin.* Liquefaction was much more likely to be observed when the body was within a coffin. On the other hand adipocere was scanty or absent in contrast to bodies buried without a coffin.
4. *Clothing at the time of burial.* The presence of clothing or some other covering was an important factor in retarding decomposition.
5. *Depth of burial.* Generally speaking, the greater the depth, the greater the preservation. In shallow graves the soil is generally well aerated, and the body subject to insect predators and animals. Furthermore, in a shallow grave, the body will be warmed in the summer months.
6. *Type of soil.* According to Mant, this factor has been overemphasised. The degree of decomposition did not vary significantly between bodies exhumed from a variety of soils. A well-drained soil was, however, conducive to mummification.
7. *Access of air to body after burial.* Continual presence of air in shallow graves has an accelerating effect on decomposition.
8. *Inclusion of something in grave.* Straw or pine lining a grave increased the rate of decomposition by supplying bacteria, acting as a heat insulator and supplying a layer of air.

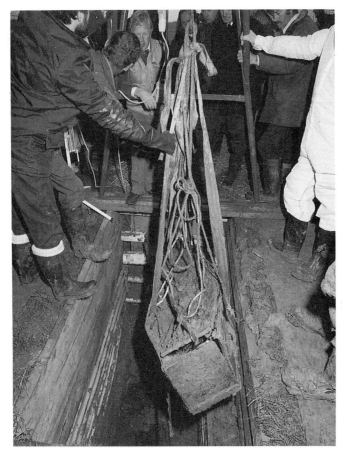

Figure 5.4(c)   Ropes were carefully passed under the coffin to secure the base. They were then attached to a pulley and lifted as shown.

Location of a death in a cold environment, such as glacier ice

Such circumstances are discussed by Ambach et al. (1991). The relationship to glacier movement is important. In such cases the scene of death and the place of discovery after a long post-mortem interval is not the same. If one knows the time after death and the place of discovery in such cases, it may be possible to ascertain the scene of death.

The account of the discovery and investigation of the 5000-year-old Neolithic 'ice man' found trapped in a glacier in the Otztaler Alps on the Austian–Italian border in a remarkable state of preservation, makes fascinating reading (Spindler,1994). He was discovered on 19 September 1991 by two mountaineers, Erika and Helmut Simon, when they spotted his head and shoulders emerging from a residual glacier in a rocky gully. A humidity band which was present on the ice man's skin, approximately 6 cm

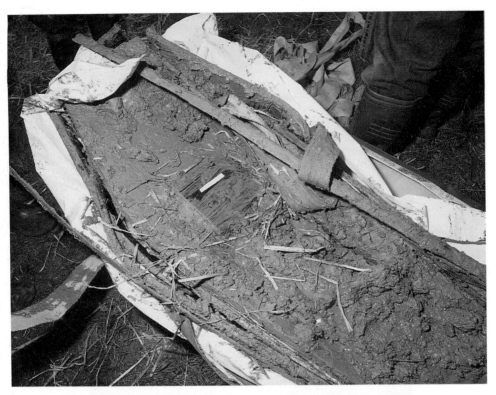

Figure 5.4(d) The coffin plate can be seen in this view, which was identified by the undertaker to the investigators. Note that, because of the poor drainage of the soil, the coffin was waterlogged and had begun to disintegrate. A great deal of care was necessary to prevent further disintegration.

wide immediately above the surface of the ice, marked the level to which the ice had melted that day between sunrise and 1.30 p.m. There had been substantial glacier ablation, the extent being on a scale that is extremely rare and occurs only in specific weather conditions. Indeed, the number of glacier bodies found during 1991 numbered six, as many as were found in the previous 39 years.

References

Ambach E., Tributsch W. and Henn R. (1991) Fatal accidents on glaciers: forensic, criminological and glaciological conclusions. *J. For. Sci.* **36**, 1469–1473.

Bruce A.H. and Rao V.J. (1991) Evaluation of dismembered human remains. *Am. J. For. Med. Pathol.* **12**, 291–299.

Camps F.E. (1962) Soil – some medico-legal aspects. In *Soil*. British Academy of Forensic Sciences, Teaching Symposium, no. 1. Sweet & Maxwell, London, pp. 47–51.

Cotton G.E., Aufderheide A.C. and Goldschmidt V.G. (1987) Preservation of human tissue immersed for five years in fresh water of known temperature. *J. For. Sci.* **32**, 1125–1130.

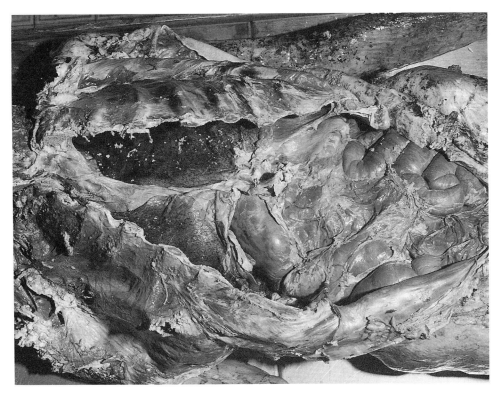

Figure 5.4(e) Internal view of the body showing reasonably good preservation of organs.

Dickinson D.J. (1977) The aerial use of an infrared camera in a police search for the body of a missing person in New Zealand. *J. For. Sci. Soc.* **16**, 205–211.

Findley P. (1948) Ignaz Philipp Semmelweiss. *Am. J. Obs. Gyn.* **55**, 700–710.

France D.L., Griffin T.J., Swanburg J.G., Lindemann J.W., Davenport G.C., Trammell V., Armbrust C.T., Kondratieff B., Nelson A., Castellano K. and Hopkins D. (1992) A multidisciplinary approach to the detection of clandestine graves. *J. For. Sci.* **37**, 1445–1458.

Gaffney C.F. and Gater J.G. (1993) Practice and method in the application of geophysical techniques in archaeology. In *Archaeological Resource Management in the UK: An Introduction*. Hunter J.R. and Ralston I.B.M. (eds). Alan Sutton, Stroud.

Gormsen H. (1972) Why have victims of death from a cold environment undressed? *Med. Sci. Law* **12**, 201–202.

Haglund W.D. and Reay D.T. (1993) Problems of recovering partial human remains at different times and locations: concerns for death investigators. *J. For. Sci.* **38**, 69–80.

Haglund W.D., Reay D.T. and Swindler D.R. (1988) Tooth mark artifacts and survival of bones in animal-scavenged human skeletons. *J. Forensic Sci.* **33**, 985–997.

Hill A.P. (1977) Disarticulation and scattering of mammalian skeletons. *Palaeopathology* **5**, 261–274.

Hunter J.R. (1994) Forensic archaeology in Britain. *Antiquity* **68**, 758–769.

Hyams B.A. and Rao V.J. (1991) Evaluation and identification of human remains. *Am. J. For. Med. Pathol.* **12**, 291–299.

Killam E.W. (1990) *The Detection of Human Remains*. Charles C. Thomas, Springfield, IL.

Kubo S. (1989) Changes in the specificity of blood groups induced by enzymes from cell fungi. *J. For. Sci.* **34**, 96–104.

Lee H.C., Gaensslen R.E., Carver H.W., Pagliaro E.M. and Carroll-Reho J. (1988) ABH antigen typing in bone tissue. *J. For. Sci.* **34**, 7–14.

Madea B. (1994) Leichenzerstuckelung mit ungewohnlicher Konservierung der Leichenteile. *Archiv Kriminol.* **193**, 72–78.

Mann R.W., Bass W.M. and Meadow L. (1990) Time since death and decomposition of the human body; variables and observations in case and experimental field studies. *J. For. Sci.* **35**, 103–111.

Mant A.K. (1953) Recent work on changes after death. In *Modern Trends in Forensic Medicine*. Simpson K. (ed.). Butterworths, London.

Mant A. and Furbank R. (1957) Adipocere – a review. *J. For. Med.* **4**, 18–35.

Mellen P.F.M., Lowry M.A. and Micozzi M.S. (1993) Experimental observations on adipocere formation. *J. For. Sci.* **38**, 91–93.

Rodriguez W.C. and Bass W.M. (1985). Decomposition of buried bodies and methods that may aid their location. *J. For. Sci.* **30**, 836–852.

Rossi M.L., Shahrom A.W., Chapman R.C. and Vanezis P. (1994) Postmortem injuries by indoor pets. *Am. J. For. Med. Pathol.* **15**, 105–109.

Simonsen J. (1977) Early formation of adipocere in temperate climate. *Med. Sci. Law* **17**, 53–55.

Sivaloganathan S. (1986) Paradoxical undressing in hypothermia. *Med. Sci. Law* **26**, 225–229.

Spindler K. (1994) *The Man in the Ice* (English translation). Weidenfeld and Nicholson, London.

Takatori T., Ishiguro N., Tarao H. and Matsumiya H. (1986) Microbial production of hydroxy and oxo fatty acids by several micro-organisms and a model of adipocere formation. *For. Sci. Int.* **32**, 5–11.

Vanezis P., Sims B.G. and Grant J. (1978) Medical and scientific investigations of an exhumation in unhallowed ground. *Med. Sci. Law* **18**, 209–221.

Wedin B, Vanggaard L., and Hirvonnen J. (1979) Paradoxical undressing in fatal hypothermia. *J. For. Sci.* **24**, 543–553.

CHAPTER 6

Entomological investigation of the scene

Introduction

Insects are extremely abundant and ubiquitous organisms. They are found almost everywhere on land and in freshwater at all times of the year, including, contrary to popular conceptions, in winter. Therefore, it is very likely that insects will be associated with dead bodies in forensically interesting situations and their presence will almost always shed light on the circumstances of a crime in a number of possible ways:

1. Time of death estimation.
2. Assessing the place of death and subsequent movement of a body to another location.
3. Occasionally, by indicating the manner of death.

Some common insects of forensic interest are shown in Figure 6.1(a)–(c).

In addition to the account given below, the reader may wish to consult the following for further information: Erzinçlioglu (1983, 1986, 1989) and Smith (1986).

Biology of flies

From the forensic point of view, flies, especially blowflies, are without doubt, the most important insects. It is essential, therefore, to give a brief introduction to their general biology in as far as is relevant to forensic situations.

The common bluebottle, *Calliphora vicina*, which belongs to the blowfly family Calliphoridae, is probably the most commonly encountered insect in forensic investigations. Like most blowflies, it requires a protein meal before it can develop its first batch of eggs. Such a meal is usually found by feeding on a body or on other sources of protein such as faeces. When mating occurs, the sperm passes into the vagina and then into three structures, known as spermathecae, via the spermathecal ducts. When the eggs are mature, they pass down the lateral oviducts and into the vagina, where they are fertilised by sperm pumped from the spermathecae. The eggs are then laid singly. Thus, fertilisation of the eggs takes place as they are being laid and not at

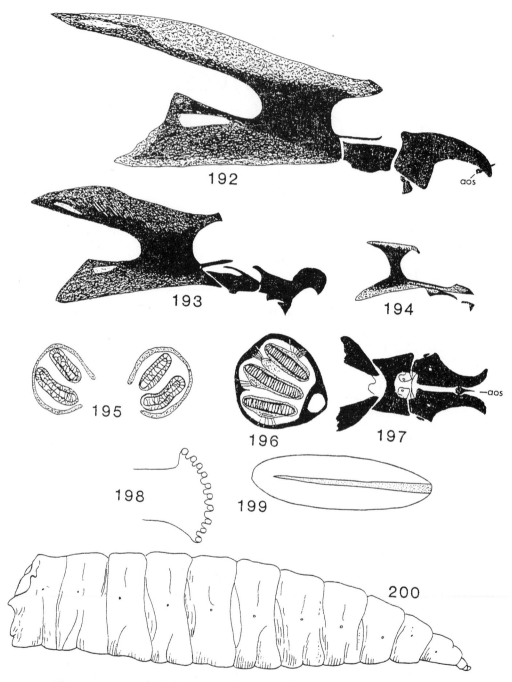

Figure 6.1(a) *Calliphora vicina* (Calliphoridae, Diptera), immature stages. Nos:
192, mouthparts, lateral third instar larva (aos = accessory oral sclerite); 193,
mouthparts, lateral, second instar larva; 194, mouthparts, lateral, first instar larva;
195, posterior spiracles, second instar larva; 196, posterior spiracles, third instar
larva; 197, mouthparts, third instar larva, ventral; 198, anterior spiracle, third instar
larva; 199, egg; 200, third instar larva, lateral (after Smith, 1986).

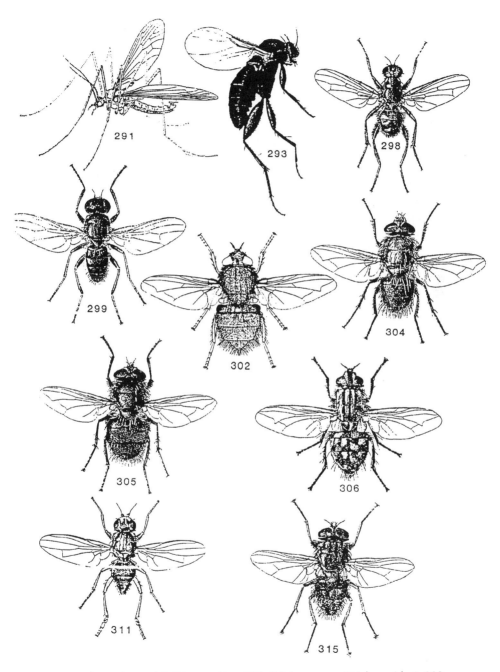

Figure 6.1(b) Adult Diptera. Nos: 291, *Trichocera* sp. (Trichoceridae); 293, *Conicera* (Phoridae, the coffin fly); 298, *Dryomyza anilis* (Dryomyzidae); 299, *Piophila casei* (Piophilidae); Calliphoridae (blowflies): 302, *Calliphora vicina* (bluebottle); 304, *Lucilia sericata* (greenbottle); 305, *Protophormia terraenovae*; 306, *Sarcophaga carnaria* (flesh-fly, Sarcophagidae); 311, *Copromyza equina* (Sphaeroceridae); 315, *Muscina stabulans* (after Smith, 1986).

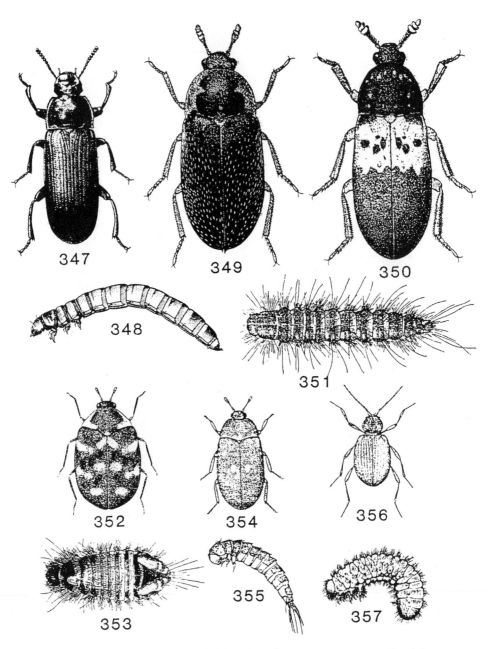

Figure 6.1(c) Coleoptera (beetles) found on dry corpses. Nos: 347, *Tenebrio molitor* (Tenebrionidae); 348, *T. molitor* larva (mealworm); 349, *Dermestes maculatus*; 350, *Dermestes lardarius*; 351, *D. lardarius* larva; 352, *Anthrenus verbasci* (Dermestidae); 353, *A. verbasci* larva; 354, *Attagenus pellio* (Dermestidae). 355, *A. pellio* larva; 356, *Ptinus tectus* (Ptinidae); 357, *P. tectus* larva (after Smith, 1986).

an earlier stage. About 300 eggs can be laid during any one bout of egg laying, and a single female may lay between 2000 and 3000 during her lifetime. After a variable period of time depending on temperature and humidity, the eggs hatch. The first instar (first stage) maggot lives for about 1 day at room temperature and then moults to the second instar (Figure 6.2), which is similarly short lived and which moults into a third instar (Figure 6.3). This is the stage that is usually met with in case work and is much longer lived than the other two stages, lasting for 5 or 6 days at room temperature. The maggot normally pupates in the soil, but in indoor conditions will pupate under carpets or bedclothes (Figure 6.4.), or even fully exposed. When pupation begins, the skin of the maggot hardens, darkens and contracts to form a barrel-shaped puparium or pupal case. The pupa develops inside the puparium. It is important not to confuse the pupa with the puparium; the latter is a protective structure while the former is the developmental stage of the insect. When development is complete, the fly breaks out of the puparium, leaving two 'caps' or opercula, and the main body of the puparium behind. The cycle then starts all over again (Figure 6.5).

In some flies, notably the fleshflies of the family Sarcophagidae, the eggs are fertilised and withheld in the body of the female inside pocket-like pouches on either side of the vagina. The eggs hatch internally and live maggots are laid on the corpse.

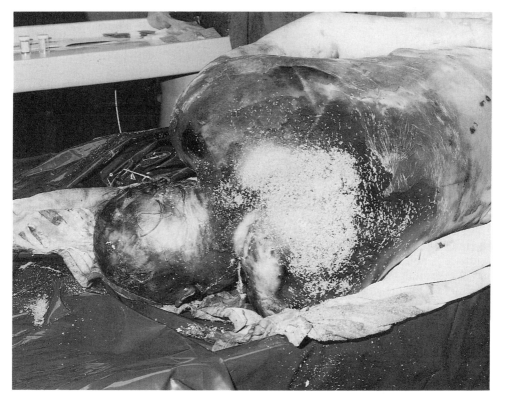

Figure 6.2 Early larval infestation (first to second instar stage) on the top of the back of a decomposing body.

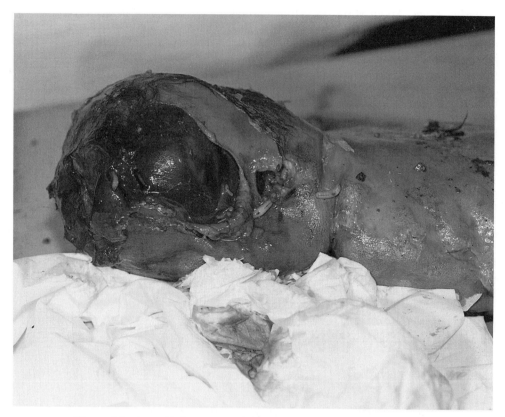

Figure 6.3   Larval infestation at the third instar stage. Note that they are particularly numerous in and around the head, which had an open wound.

Entomological examination of the body

The entomological examination of the body, although the province of the forensic entomologist, is best carried out in conjunction with the pathologist, so that other evidence is not disturbed. The natural body orifices, i.e., eyes, ears, mouth, nose, anus and the genital region, and any wounds that may be present, must be examined carefully for the presence of maggots. Fly eggs, newly hatched blowfly maggots and the full-grown maggots of smaller fly species, may be very small, and a lens may be needed during the examination. A lens that can be worn over the eye, or held in the eye, is particularly useful, as it leaves both hands free to carry out the examination. There are also special lenses that can be fitted onto spectacles. A fine forceps and fine paint brush must be at hand for removing larval specimens; the smaller specimens are best removed with a wetted brush, as they can be damaged easily.

It is often the case that larvae will burrow deeply into the tissues and may be found deep inside the throat, the nasal cavities, etc. It is therefore advisable to be in attendance with the pathologist whilst he is carrying out his post-mortem examination,

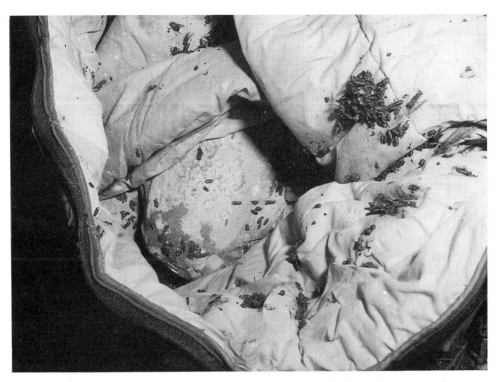

Figure 6.4   The pupal stage of infestation. Note that the larvae have pupated within the coverings in which the body had been wrapped. A few adult flies are also seen.

in order to be able to take further samples when they appear. After the examination of the orifices and wounds, a general examination of the body should be carried out. Any insects crawling upon the body should be collected using forceps, or in the case of larger insects (e.g., beetles, etc.), a large tube or jar can be used to capture the specimen. A fine comb may be used to remove specimens from the hair of the deceased. An examination of any marks on the body should be made, especially if they seem to have a patterned appearance, since such marks may have been caused by insect bites or secretions, but may initially be mistaken for evidence of wilful post-mortem mutilation. Photographs and sketches of such marks are useful for detailed examination later. Large flying insects, e.g., flies or moths, may be difficult to catch with forceps or tubes, but may be caught relatively easily with a small hand net. Finally, any clothes on the body must be removed and searched for insect specimens. In addition, if the body is transported back to the mortuary in a body bag, a search for any insects in the bag when the body is removed may prove fruitful, since very small insects that may have gone undetected during the post-mortem examination may be found at a later stage.

A very important aspect of forensic entomology is temperature measurement at the scene. This is because temperature is the single most important factor governing the rate of development of maggots. Therefore, knowledge of the temperature at which the maggots were developing is indispensable where estimating larval age is

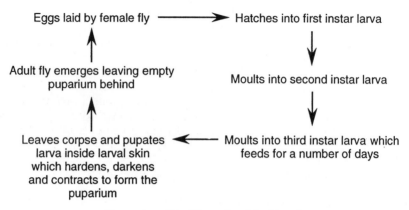

Figure 6.5   The life cycle of the blowfly.

concerned. The temperature of the body, especially the actual mass of the maggots in the body *must* be taken. The ambient temperature must also be measured. For all these purposes, an ordinary mercury thermometer is not very suitable, but an electronic thermometer with a thermocouple or temperature probe attached is ideal. The thermocouple or probe can be inserted deep into the tissues and an accurate temperature reading can be taken. An air probe may be used for measuring the ambient temperature.

Collection and preservation of the specimens

During examination and collection of specimens, maggots, flies, beetles and tineid caterpillars are best placed immediately in tubes of acetic alcohol (3 parts 70 per cent ethanol: 1 part glacial acetic acid). If no preservative fluid is available and, as a last resort, killing of specimens may be done by immersion in very hot water. The method is not recommended however, as it damages some of the internal structures that need to be examined in the laboratory. Tineid moths are best collected and taken back to the laboratory alive, since immersion in fluid results in the loss of the wing scales, which are useful features in identification. Moths can be caught and placed in dry tubes; a piece of cotton wool should then be pushed into the jar in order to restrict the movements of the insect. Some specimens should be kept alive, if possible, especially examples of blowfly maggots. Such specimens may be placed in a jar with some tissue and sawdust; the lid of the jar should be perforated to allow gaseous exchange. Live specimens must be transported into the laboratory as quickly as possible.

In the case of maggot-infested corpses, it is necessary to collect fairly large, representative samples of maggots. What constitutes a large sample will, of course, depend on the degree of infestation, but two jars of maggots can usually be regarded as adequate. The reason for taking large samples is that this makes it possible to interpret the population of maggots more confidently. On any maggot-infested body, a number of different-sized maggots will be found; some of the smaller ones will have been derived from eggs laid later than the eggs that produced the larger maggots.

Thus it is usually more useful to concentrate on the larger maggots, although there are pitfalls in doing this as well. As described above, the eggs of many blowflies are fertilised during egg laying, but it often happens that one egg, and only one, is fertilised earlier. This happens because the length of the vagina can accommodate only one egg and the first egg to pass down the oviduct will be fertilised before the others. This egg, however, may not be laid immediately, if the fly has not found a corpse to lay its eggs on; it will develop inside the fly and when egg laying takes place, it will be at a more advanced stage of development than all the other eggs laid during that bout of egg laying. It will therefore hatch first. Thus, there is often a small number of rather large maggots and a vastly larger number of smaller maggots on the body. It is clear that these large maggots will give a misleading time of death estimate, since they had been developing before the fly arrived at the body; they therefore need to be identified as being what they are and a large sample will help to do this.

Labelling of the specimens is important. With fluid-preserved specimens, a label written in pencil (not ink) should be inserted inside the tube with the specimens. It should have details of where on the body the specimens were collected and preserved. This latter point is important because the minimum time of death estimation is arrived at by working backwards from the time the maggots themselves were killed.

In an indoor location, after examination of the body, a general entomological examination of the room in which the body is lying should be made. If the body is lying on a bed, the bed clothes should be searched for insects, especially the puparia, or pupal cases, of flies. Empty puparia and puparia from which the flies have not yet emerged should be placed in tubes, without preservative fluid, and kept in place by means of a cotton wool plug. The carpet and general surroundings should also be searched and samples taken. If there are any items of blood-stained clothing lying in the room, an examination of these should be made and any insects present sampled.

If the body is lying in a car or other vehicle, an examination of this should be made. The exterior of the car must also be examined, since minute insects are often found adhering to the car and these may give evidence as to where the car may have been. The grooves around the windscreen and headlights should receive special attention.

In an outdoor location, if the body is lying on the soil, soil samples should be taken from underneath the body and kept in large specimen bags. No preservative should be added. Since the soil fauna beneath the body will change with time when the body is resting on the surface, analysis of the fauna present at a given time will give an indication of how long the body had been lying in that position. Generally speaking, the soil fauna (both number of species and number of individuals) will drop dramatically to a particular minimum point, after which a new fauna, with increasing numbers of species and individuals will develop (Figure 6.6). In order to analyse the soil fauna meaningfully, it is necessary to have control samples taken at some distance from the body, but from equivalent depths. A description of the habitat and its prevailing vegetation should be made, and temperature measurements of the body, soil and air, taken. Further temperature records for the area may be obtained from the nearest meteorological office. Photographs of outdoor scenes are particularly valuable for the interpretation of entomological data.

The method of examination of an exhumed body for entomological purposes is essentially the same as that for any other body. However, it is also important to search the coffin for any insects (especially fly puparia) and, if possible, to take samples of the wood of the coffin for closer inspection back in the laboratory. The insects inhabiting

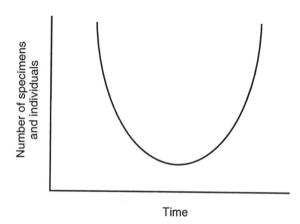

Figure 6.6   A graph showing that the fauna in a soil under a body will decrease to a particularly low level, then a different fauna will develop with a corresponding increase.

the wood may themselves reveal useful information. In the case of uncoffined bodies, the soil surrounding the body must be sampled, especially the soil underneath the body. Control samples from equivalent depths away from the body should also be taken for comparison.

In cases where the body is immersed in water, the body should be examined for any sign of freshwater invertebrates. This means a painstaking examination of the body from end to end. Samples of hair and skin may be taken, and preserved in alcohol for subsequent laboratory examination. During the examination of the body, any evidence of feeding by fish should also be looked for.

Time of death estimation

First and most commonly, the maggots (or blowfly larvae) that are often found infesting a corpse, may give an estimate of time of death. In such cases a minimum time of death estimate based on larval age is made. It is clear that the body cannot have been dead for a time that is less than the age of the maggots. In other words, if it is estimated that the maggots on the corpse are 5 days old, the deceased could not have died with a post-mortem interval of less than 5 days, although the body may well have been dead for a lot longer than that. The age of the maggots therefore can give a minimum estimate of the post-mortem interval. For an *actual* time of death estimate, further evidence is needed. Since blowflies will arrive at a corpse and lay eggs on it within an hour or two after death if the body is exposed during the warmer months of the year, the minimum time of death estimate is effectively the actual time of death. This holds true if it assumed that the body had been exposed (i.e., not concealed in such a way that would prevent the flies from having access to it) since death. Generally speaking, burying a body, or placing it in a sealed body bag or in a container with a tightly fitting lid would result in effective concealment of a body from blowfly activity, but simply hiding a body under layers of sheets or under vegetation would not. It must be emphasised that what constitutes effective conceal-ment may depend very much on the prevailing circumstances of the case. An accurate description of the scene is therefore important if accurate conclusions are to be drawn.

Low temperatures below about 10 °C will prevent the activity (i.e., the flight, egg laying, etc.) of blowflies. Therefore, if a body is lying fully exposed at such temperatures, blowflies will not lay eggs on it until the temperature rises. A time of death estimation made on the basis of larval age in such a case will therefore give a minimum time of death that will be less than the actual time of death. However, it is interesting to note that, while adult fly activity ceases at around 10 °C, the maggots can remain active at much lower temperatures, even at high sub-zero temperatures for certain periods of time. At sub-zero temperatures, maggots may remain active, but will die sooner or later, depending on the exact temperature and the length of time they are exposed to it. Knowledge of the thermal biology of flies and maggots can be applied very usefully in cases of this sort. In one case it was possible to conclude, on the basis of climatic data supplied by the local meteorological office, that the presence of maggots on a body exposed in the open indicated that death had, in fact, taken place indoors. This is because the temperatures on the days prior to discovery of the body were too cold for blowfly activity and because the period of time at these low temperatures was too long for the maggots to have survived them. In other words, the maggots on the body could not have survived from an early bout of egg laying prior to the onset of the cold weather. The presence of maggots on the body indicated that egg laying had occurred indoors and that the body had been subsequently deposited out of doors.

When attempting to determine time of death on the basis of maggot age it is important that the species of maggot be identified. This is because different species develop at different rates and it is knowledge of the rate of development at different temperatures that is used to determine the age of the maggot.

A large number of cases in which time of death was determined entomologically are on record. However, it sometimes happens that maggots are absent from a body when one would have expected them to be present if a given account of events was true. The absence of insects from such a situation instantly gives rise to doubts as to the veracity of the statement. In one documented case, the accused claimed that the body had been lying in an exposed location during the height of the summer for over 2 months. The absence of maggots from the body and the absence of any evidence that maggots had ever fed upon the body suggested that he was lying. This was shown to be the case on the basis of other evidence.

Another means of determining time of death, especially in cases where death has clearly occurred months or years prior to discovery, is by an analysis of the whole assemblage of insect species that are found on the corpse at the time of discovery. Since the species composition of the corpse fauna will change as decomposition progresses with time, the identification of the species found at a given time may give an indication of time of death. This concept, while very straightforward in theory, is not at all straightforward in practice. A faunal succession of this kind will always take place on a body but it is virtually impossible to predict what that succession will be in any given situation. Tables of the faunal succession often appear in forensic and entomological publications; these are of no use whatsoever, since they are simply a record of events that have taken place on a given occasion. Since the insect fauna will differ between localities, seasons and many other factors, it is not possible to say at the outset what form the succession is likely to take. Attempts at distilling a generalised picture of the faunal succession also fail because our knowledge of what attracts insects at different times is far from complete. This does not mean that the phenomenon of succession is of no use in forensic investigations. Indeed, it can be of great use if an analysis of the insect fauna on the body is conducted cautiously. The following is an example of an actual case in which the phenomenon of the faunal succession was used to good effect.

CASE 6.1
The body of an elderly woman was discovered in her house at the end of October. A large number of small flies belonging to the species *Leptocera caenosa* was found on the body. These were present as adult flies, maggots and pupal cases, some of which contained pupae and others of which were empty. Four other species of related small flies were found on the body, but were represented by empty pupal cases only. In other words, four other species had been active on the body at an earlier time, but were now only represented by their non-living remains. Knowledge of the seasonality and behaviour of these four species led to the conclusion that death had occurred much earlier in the year than was originally supposed. In this case it was possible to use the faunal succession to arrive at useful conclusions. Many other such cases are on record.

Assessment of place of death

The second kind of information that an entomological examination may bring to light is evidence concerning *place* of death. Since so many insect species are specific to certain ecological habitats or geographical areas, the presence of an insect on a corpse lying outside the natural habitat or geographical area can give convincing evidence, not only that the body had been moved but where it had been moved from. Note that the word 'place' has two meanings in this context; a geographical meaning and an ecological one. An ecological place is a habitat: a woodland, a house, a suburban garden, a seashore, etc. A geographical place is an actual locality: London, the north of Scotland, south Wales or the island of Jersey. Knowledge of both the geographical distribution and ecological preferences of an insect can often result in a fairly accurate description of where the body had been lying before it was moved to the locality in which it was discovered.

Assisting with manner of death

Insect evidence may shed light on manner of death in some cases. Manner of death is primarily the province of the pathologist, but occasionally the entomologist may be able to contribute to the resolution of this problem, especially in cases where extensive decomposition has taken place. Blowflies normally lay their eggs in the natural body orifices (eyes, ears, nose, mouth, anus). This is because these areas are usually moist and shaded, reducing the risk of desiccation to the eggs. If an open wound is present on the body it will be perceived by the flies as yet another orifice and will attract them to lay eggs in it. The maggots in such a case will be distributed on the body in a very different pattern from the usual pattern arising from eggs laid only in the natural body orifices and will thus give an idea of the locations of wounds that are no longer detectable themselves.

Finally, it is worth noting that almost any insect found at the scene may contribute some information to the reconstruction of events. Insects account for about 80 per cent of all known animal species. It follows from this that each species is very specialised in its life habits, distribution, etc. Therefore, from the forensic point of view, any insect species will shed light on *some* aspect of events.

References

Erzinçlioglu Y.Z. (1983) The application of entomology to forensic medicine. *Med. Sci. Law* **23**, 57–63.

Erzinçlioglu Y.Z. (1986) Areas of research in forensic entomology. *Med. Sci. Law* **26**, 273–278.

Erzinçlioglu Y.Z. (1989) Entomology, zoology and forensic science: the need for expansion. *For. Sci. Int.* **43**, 209–213.

Smith K.G.V. (1986) *A Manual of Forensic Entomology*. British Museum (Natural History), London, and Cornell University Press.

PART 2

Scene Types

CHAPTER 7

Scene type: firearm deaths

The investigation of a suspected shooting scene ideally involves the specialist firearms expert working side by side with the rest of the investigation team at the scene as well as being present later on at the autopsy. This expert's assistance at the scene is invaluable and indispensable.

In a shooting incident there will invariably be a greater or lesser amount of blood and its distribution will be the province of the biologist specially trained to interpret any blood patterns (see Chapter 4).

As with all types of scenes, the prerequisite before anything is touched, apart from the doctor certifying death, is the recording of the incident by adequate photography. As well as general views, close-ups should be taken that show any obvious wounds, associated blood and, particularly with firearm scenes, the relative positions of any weapon and/or bullet holes and cartridge cases. It is well documented that some considerable physical activity can follow after shooting, which makes accurate recording of the scene important (DiMaio, 1985).

Types of weapon encountered

Outside the military environment and in the occasional politically motivated incident, it is unusual to encounter weapons other than handguns and shotguns. The various categories of firearms are briefly considered as well as the nature of the evidence to be found at a scene in relation to each type.

HANDGUNS

These may be subdivided into two main types, the pistol and the revolver. Both are designed to be fired with one hand but they have major differences, which affect the evidence potentially retrievable at the scene.

Pistols

The pistol can be a single-shot weapon, although the more frequently encountered type is the self-loading or semi-automatic type. The term 'automatic' is often applied to this type of gun, but this is a misnomer as it is strictly limited to the sub-machine gun and machine gun, which are described briefly below.

The pistol therefore in its popular configuration is a single-barrelled weapon, firing a single bullet through a rifled barrel. It is provided with a magazine, normally housed in the grip, which holds the rounds of ammunition. In a small pocket pistol of 0.22", 0.25" and 0.32" calibres, the magazine capacity will be in the region of 7–8 rounds whereas in the larger calibres of 9 mm and 0.45", and with modern designs, the magazine capacity may be as many as 18 rounds.

As mentioned above, the pistol under consideration is a self-loading weapon. After cocking the action and loading the first round into the chamber the gun is ready to fire. Pressure on the trigger of some 5–10 pounds will fire this first round and discharge the bullet. What happens next depends on the mechanism of the gun in question.

In the conventional weapon the recoil force generated by the discharge of the cartridge will cycle the mechanism 'automatically' and eject the fired cartridge case clear of the gun. Recoil is an ever-present phenomenon of gun discharge. The principle is enshrined in Newton's Third Law of Motion, which states that 'every action has an equal and opposite reaction'. Therefore, once the bullet starts to move at relatively high velocity, so the gun tries to move backwards at the same rate. It cannot of course, because it is much heavier than the bullet and it is generally well supported by the hand. The action, however, does move backwards relative to the body of the pistol and takes the cartridge case with it, carried on the extractor. Towards the rear of its travel, this case is struck by the ejector and thrown clear, thus generating a potential piece of evidence for the scene examiner. The return spring in the pistol will then exert itself and the action will run forward again, taking the next cartridge from the magazine, leaving the weapon cocked and ready for a further pull on the trigger to fire the next shot.

In the second type of pistol mechanism, the high-pressure gases generated within the cartridge and barrel are utilised to drive a piston rearward, and cycle the action rather than just the recoil energy. This 'gas operation' is far more commonplace in modern military rifles and machine guns, although a few pistols use it. The end result is the same, with a fired cartridge case ejected at the scene, sometimes several yards away from the gun.

Revolvers

This is the second major category of handgun. Again it is a repeating weapon but with the rounds of ammunition held in separate chambers within a revolving cylinder. By far the most common configuration is six rounds, although with small calibres, capacities of up to 12 are sometimes seen.

Most revolvers can be fired in two ways: single action, where the exposed hammer is first cocked and a relatively light trigger pull in the region of 3–5 pounds applied; or double action, where a long heavy pull, perhaps of some 12–20 pounds is applied to the trigger, which both cocks the action and advances the cylinder one chamber prior to allowing the hammer to drop and fire the gun.

The important difference between the pistol and the revolver is that, with the revolver the fired cartridge case remains within the chamber and is not ejected into the scene.

As stated above, both pistols and revolvers discharge a single bullet. Although there are exceptions to every rule, generally speaking the pistol will fire a jacketed bullet, whereas the revolver bullet is often plain lead. The jacket is a covering of a tough cupro-nickel, steel or brass over the lead core, designed to protect the soft lead from the violent actions of the loading cycle. While most bullets are designed to remain intact in the body, it is often the case that, if bone is struck or the bullet exits from the body and goes on to strike a hard surface, the core and the jacket will separate and be located separately at the scene.

CASE 7.1
The author has investigated a shooting incident where a jacketed bullet separated on entry to a second person, having passed through the elbow and across the back of the person aimed at. The bullet jacket was found some distance from the line of fire and it was not until the jacket was examined closely in the laboratory that it was discovered that fibres from the outer clothing were adhering, as a result of it having been carried for some distance on the sleeve of the robber's clothing in his attempt to escape.

SHOTGUNS

This is the major type of weapon encountered in everyday crime. It differs fundamentally from the handgun in that it has a smooth-bored barrel and it fires a charge of pellets (shot) propelled by wadding. In a typical 12-bore cartridge, there will be around 300 pellets, which are potentially retrievable at the scene.

The shotgun in its unmodified state is a large weapon, designed to be fired from the shoulder and typically with a barrel of some 26–30 inches (65–75 cm) in length. It is rare for a gun such as this to be used outside the domestic environment, as the sheer size makes it difficult to conceal. The answer therefore is to 'saw it off', and the result is a much shorter weapon with a barrel of some 12–14 inches (30–35 cm) and the stock reduced to little more than a pistol-type grip.

Shortening a shotgun in this way has two main consequences apart from ease of concealment:

1. The perceived recoil is intensified because of the lighter weight.
2. At a given distance the shot charge will spread to a greater extent than from the original barrel because the choke has been removed.

As with the location of any bullets at a scene the identification of pellet impact must be undertaken carefully. The location of a partial pattern, perhaps associated with a blood distribution, will be a very good pointer as to where the victim was at the time of shooting. Following measurement and scale photography of the pellet pattern, the scene investigator should attempt to retrieve a selection of pellets for subsequent laboratory analysis.

At short distances, the wadding will travel with the shot charge, and it can cause wounding and damage in its own right. There are two main types of wadding, the card/felt and the relatively recent plastic. The first type can be difficult to find if outdoors in rough terrain. However, the plastic type is usually distinctive in appearance and not readily confused with normal environmental debris. As mentioned above, wadding will travel with the shot for a few feet before falling away and it is common for the wadding to be retrieved at post-mortem together with pellets when the range of firing is short.

Shotguns come in all shapes and sizes from single and double-barrelled sporting guns through to pump action and other repeating designs with magazine capacities of up to nine cartridges. In a scene with multiple shots discharged, cartridge cases may be ejected from the shotgun in a similar way to the pistol and their position at the scene will give a good indication as to the position of the person shooting the gun.

MACHINE GUNS AND MILITARY RIFLES

As was mentioned earlier in the chapter, military weapons are seldom encountered in crime on the mainland of the United Kingdom outside politically motivated incidents and those involving military personnel.

The modern military rifle with its close relation, the machine pistol, or sub-machine gun, differs in one major aspect from the shotguns and handguns referred to above. They are invariably selective-fire weapons; that is to say they will fire in a single-shot fashion in just the same way as a self-loading pistol but they have the additional capacity to discharge in a 'fully-automatic' fashion, where missiles continue to be discharged, until the trigger is released or the magazine is empty.

A typical modern military weapon will have a magazine capacity of 25–30 rounds and a cyclic rate in the region of 400–600 rounds per minute, so will empty in approximately 3 seconds of continuous fire. As with ejected cases from the self-loading pistol and shotgun, the careful analysis of their distribution is very important. Of particular significance will be the distribution of the bullet impacts, the position of which will, if the gun is in automatic mode, alter as the recoil angle increases.

Recoil

In the vast majority of weapons, the barrel will be situated above the grip and so when the gun discharges, the recoil force acting along the barrel sets up a turning moment along the grip, or butt-stock, the result being that the muzzle rises. As it rises in automatic fire, then this turning moment gets increasingly larger and, unless in the hands of an experienced shooter, the gun will rapidly climb away out of control with potentially disasterous consequences.

In the case of self-inflicted or accidental gunshot wounds with the weapon still at the scene, the position of the gun relative to the body must be noted carefully and the distance from the body considered. Whilst it is not uncommon for the deceased to remain holding a handgun, the violent recoil of a shotgun, particularly if sawn-off, can propel the weapon some distance from the body. In a case known to the author involving a single-barrelled sawn-off 12-bore shotgun to the head, the recoil sent the weapon some 3 metres from the body.

Ricochet bullet marks

Crime scenes, where bullets have ricocheted, will generally leave traces of metal from the projectile, whether bullet or pellet, which can be readily identified in the laboratory (Burke and Rowe, 1992). In addition, the surface may be damaged by the projectile producing a crater in the wall or by gouging out part of the surface. The nature of the damage sustained will depend to a great extent on the type of surface. For example, elongated gouge marks, extending in the long axis of the direction of the projectile, will appear elongated in a soft metal surface (Mitosinka, 1971; Janssen and Levine, 1982) or plasterboard (Jordan et al., 1988). The width of the gouge marks will indicate the diameter of the projectile. On the other hand, ricochet marks in soil or sand will be less well defined (Haag, 1975). Projectiles may pick up trace evidence from surfaces and a scanning electron microscope can be used to identify particles. In the case described by DiMaio et al. (1987) limestone was detected, which had originated from a stone surface from which the bullet had ricocheted.

Mode of death – homicide, suicide or accident

In the vast majority of cases, there is little doubt as to the mode of causation of the fatal wounding. However, in some, the distinction is not so clear and one must therefore always approach each case with an open and enquiring mind. Careful examination of the scene, together with the pathological findings elicited at the post-mortem examination will, in many cases where there may be initial doubt, enable one to reach the correct conclusion. Pathological factors that need to be taken into account include the site of the wound or wounds, their multiplicity, range, signs of a struggle on the body, dexterity of the victim (left- or right-handedness), residues on hands and injuries on the hand from the firing weapon.

At the scene, consideration should be given to the presence or absence of a weapon, and its position in relation to the body, position of blood stains, signs of a disturbance, accessibility to the scene (e.g., whether and how the door was secured from the inside), position of spent cartridge cases, trajectory of missiles, and impact marks on objects or surfaces from missiles and their distribution.

The site of the wound in most suicide cases conforms to well-recognised selected sites such as the temple, mouth, and midline structures to the front of the body. The direction of the wound track from the site is a further good indication of the aim of the deceased towards a particular vital structure such as the heart or brain.

The range of discharge of the firearm is another useful factor, which may help confirm or negate death as being self-inflicted. Unless there is some mechanism to discharge a firearm from a distance further than arm's reach, then such a discharge is extremely unlikely to have been self-inflicted. Gerdin (1980) related the case of a 77-year-old man who had contrived to ensure that the pistol, which he used to kill himself, was thrown aside by the elasticity of a rubber band, to which it was tied, and was thereby hidden. After the shot the man fell and crushed his head, which initially concealed the bullet wound. An investigation of the scene between the various experts involved, revealed the true circumstances. No explanation for the attempt to conceal the suicide was found.

In the following case, the position of the body at the scene, together with the distribution of blood staining and position of the weapon enabled a confident assumption of suicide to be made.

CASE 7.2
An elderly male was found dead at home with a double-barrelled 12-bore shotgun by the left side of his body. Blood was sprayed over the ceiling and wall behind the deceased as shown in Figure 7.1(a). Closer examination of the body revealed a shotgun

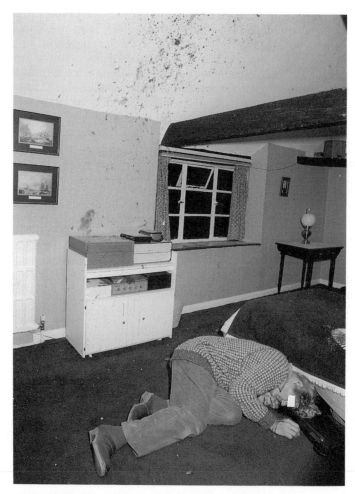

Figure 7.1(a)   The deceased is shown in the bedroom by the side of his bed. To his right side is a double-barrelled 12-bore shotgun. Blood spattering is clearly seen on the wall and ceiling behind him.

entry wound to the right temple (Figure 7.1(b)). Live cartridge cases were found scattered in an adjoining room. The position of the blood staining clearly indicated that the weapon had been fired from below upwards with the muzzle of the gun pressed against his right temple.

The position of the weapon in relation to the body should always be examined with

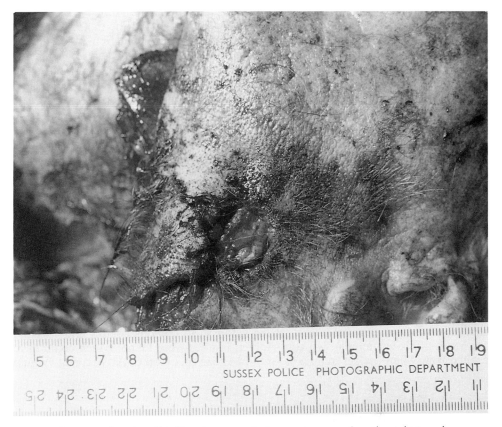

Figure 7.1(b)   A self-inflicted contact shotgun entry wound on the right temple.

care when assessing whether or not the deceased could have fired the weapon. The following is an example of a simulated suicide.

CASE 7.3
A young female, was found with a 0.22 semi-automatic rifle by her right side and two wounds in her neck (one being only a flesh wound). It was at first thought that she had killed herself after she had killed her two children, mother and father. Sometime later, however, a silencer was retrieved from the gun cupboard with blood on the inside, the outside having been wiped. The brother was arrested and convicted of murdering all five members of his family.

The latter case illustrates the need for comprehensive scene examination and maintaining a low threshold of suspicion in all cases, particularly where multiple deaths are involved.

Shooting oneself whilst driving a motor car has been encountered occasionally, and careful examination of the vehicle and the crash site will reveal the true nature of events. When one is called to a fatal 'road traffic accident' it is important to bear in mind, particularly if one is dealing with a single vehicle occupant and there are no clear eye-witness accounts of the circumstances of the crash, that there may be some other mode of death, other than injuries received from vehicular impact. Diligent examination of the vehicle and the scene is vital because the collision damage to the vehicle may overlay any damage caused by projectiles. Furthermore, there may be secondary injuries to the deceased, particularly burns, which may obscure a gunshot wound. The examiner will also need to establish from where the gun was fired, i.e., from within or from outside the vehicle and also whether or not there were other occupants in the car other than the deceased. Murphy (1989) gives an account of a vehicular suicidal shooting in a young woman. Her car was seen to leave the road, became airborne and came to rest on its roof. Initially it was felt to have been a road traffic accident. On closer inspection when the vehicle was righted, a 0.357 revolver was found on the ground beside the car. A single fatal self-inflicted gunshot wound was found in the centre of the chest and a suicide note in her purse.

CASE 7.4

A 25-year-old man was found slumped on the front passenger side of his Ford Anglia estate car, which had veered off the road and landed in a field by a ditch some way from the highway. The police were informed of an incident where a man had been firing a gun indiscriminately from within his car whilst driving, at other passing cars, causing damage to the mini saloon as shown in Figure 7.2(a), fortunately, not causing any serious injury to the occupant. The driver of the Ford Anglia then turned the gun on himself. His car then veered off the road and landed in a ditch after crashing through a fence. After removal of the deceased from the car, a revolver was found in the well of the passenger side and, at the autopsy, an obvious contact entry wound was noted to his left temple. No ante-mortem injuries were found, which could have resulted from blunt impact trauma as would be seen in a road traffic accident (Figure 7.2(b)–(e)).

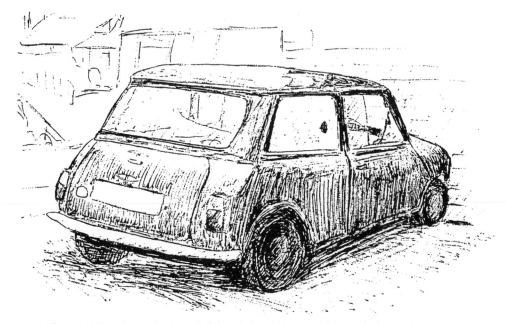

Figure 7.2(a)   A mini saloon (left-hand drive) showing shattered glass to both side windows on the right-hand side caused by two bullet impacts.

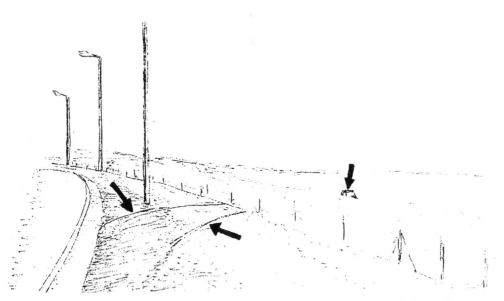

Figure 7.2(b)   A view of the location where the deceased's vehicle left the road. Two wheel marks are clearly seen going from the verge of the highway towards the fence.

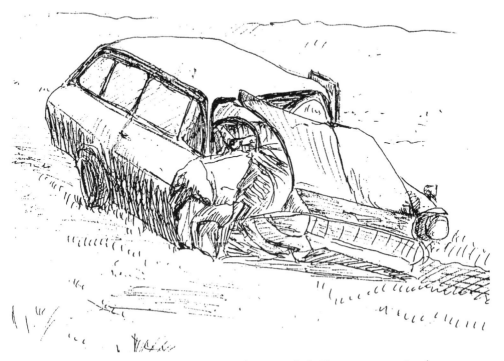

Figure 7.2(c)   The deceased's Ford Anglia car in ditch. There was extensive damage to the front of the car.

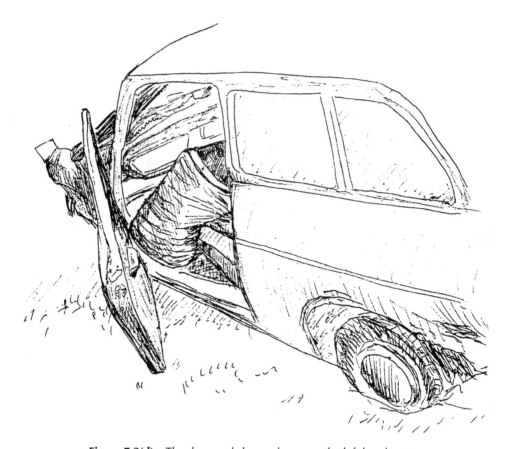

Figure 7.2(d)   The deceased slumped over on the left-hand seat.

Accidental gunshot fatalities require careful consideration of the circumstances surrounding the incident, thorough inspection of the scene and obviously examination of the firearm concerned in order to test the validity of accidental discharge.

Copeland (1984) studied gunshot injuries over a period of 11 years (1972–1982) and found that there were 54 due to accidental injury (0.143 per cent of all firearm fatalities during this period). He pointed out that consideration of the scene circumstances was just as important as the autopsy findings.

The case described below concerns an accidental fatality in a farm manager.

CASE 7.5
A 62-year-old male was found sitting in his tractor in the middle of a field. He was slumped over the steering wheel as shown in Figure 7.3(a). The tractor engine was switched off and both doors were shut. He had apparently been having problems with pigeons and had taken the gun with him to scare them away. It would appear that the deceased had the gun in the cab of his tractor and had either reached down to pick it up, or it fell over and he bent down to retrieve it. In doing so, the gun discharged causing a fatal injury to the right side of his lower chest (Figure 7.3(b)). From the character of the

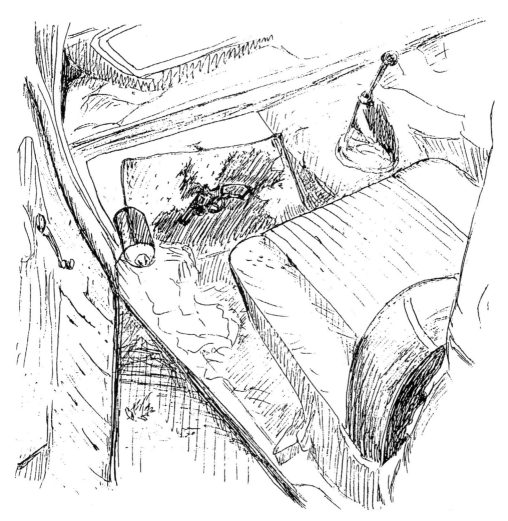

Figure 7.2(e) A close-up of the front passenger side showing a revolver lying on the foot mat. There is also extensive blood staining in the same area, from where the deceased's head had been lying.

wound, the gun appeared to have discharged from about under half a metre from the deceased. The gun then fell out of the vehicle and was run over by the tractor and found 12 metres behind the vehicle (Figure 7.3(c)). The deceased then apparently managed to turn the ignition off.

In a case described by Dix et al. (1991) a man was found guilty of killing his wife, although her body was never found. Her car contained fragments of bone (identified as skull), glass, shotgun pellets and dried blood. DNA fingerprinting was used to establish the victim's identity. From the evidence found, it was shown that the defendant's wife had received a fatal shotgun injury in her car.

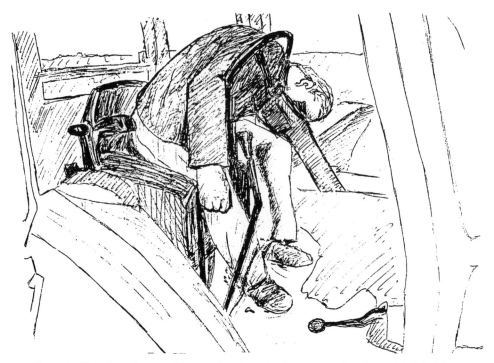

Figure 7.3(a)   The deceased is seated in the cab of his tractor, leaning to his left side after receiving a fatal wound to his right side.

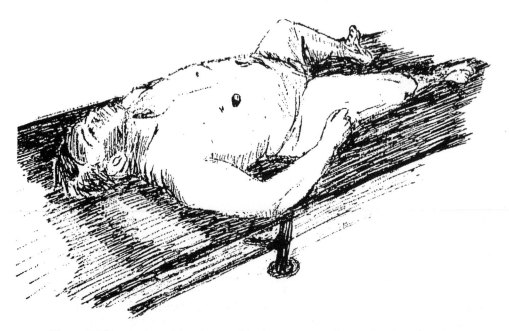

Figure 7.3(b)   A view of the deceased in the mortuary, after undressing, showing the fatal wound on the right side of the chest.

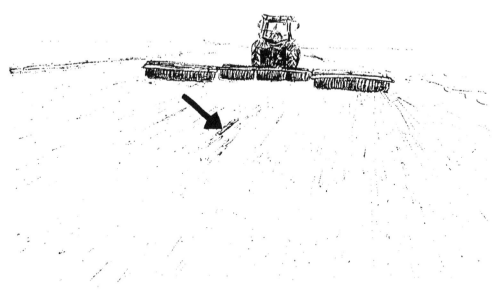

Figure 7.3(c)   The gun is shown lying about 12 metres behind the tractor. Following the line of the soil furrows, it is clear that it is on the right side of the tractor, consistent with it falling out of the cab from that side.

Scene reconstruction

It is essential in all suspicious as well as obvious homicide cases, to examine and preserve where appropriate, all the available trace evidence to assist the investigator in establishing a case against any perpetrators. A necessary part of such an investigation is the accurate reconstruction of events, which aims to provide valuable information about trajectories (Roberts and Hanby, 1985), position of victim(s) and firing position of gunman (Nennstiel, 1985) and their various movements.

For example, a thorough scene examination should be carried out to ascertain: the number, location and damage produced by missiles; distribution of spent cartridge cases, wadding, etc.; scattered debris produced by damage from impacts to structures such as walls, glass, wood, etc.; position of blood spattering and position of body tissues found at the scene. All such findings, when considered in the light of information provided by the pathologist, such as the site of entry and exit wounds, and their relative positions on the body, ricochet injuries, approximate estimation of range and so on, should allow a reasonable attempt to be made at reconstructing events.

Reay et al. (1986), describe how they were able to reconstruct a shooting scene in which 13 people were killed because they were immobilised before being shot. The victims were patrons of an oriental gambling club and were murdered systematically during a robbery. Each of the victims was tied with a ligature with their hands and feet behind their back (hog tied), robbed and then shot. They were thus able to assess the trajectories of the gunshot wounds and approximate position of the weapon at the time of firing. They found that initially shots were fired from a distance of some 6 metres away from the victims, from a slightly elevated platform. Furthermore, by assessing the location of ejected casings, they were also able to say that shots were fired as the perpetrators walked among the victims. The one survivor was able to corroborate this reconstruction.

CASE 7.6

A further example of trajectory reconstruction from scene examination was provided following the shooting of a police officer outside a diplomatic mission (Figure 7.4(a) and (b)).

Shots had been fired from the mission towards a group of demonstrators who were controlled by police behind a line of linked metal barriers. One bullet struck and killed the police officer in question.

The pathological findings relating to the injury were of prime importance at an early stage in the investigation and enabled the pathologist to demonstrate a downward angle through the chest and arm of between 60° and 70° to the horizontal plane.

Because of the nature of the incident, the scene could not be examined immediately. However, the square in which the mission was situated was sealed off, thus effectively preserving the scene.

Eventual examination of the barriers and pavement areas in front of the mission revealed bullets and fragments, and directional impact marks could be seen.

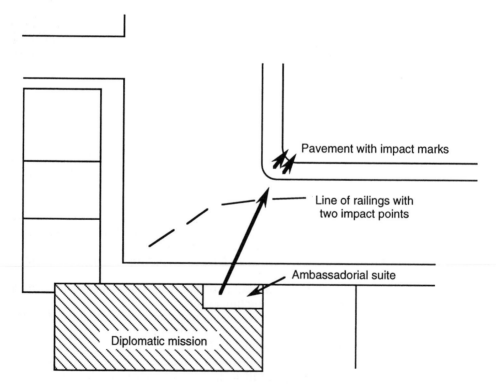

Figure 7.4(a)   A view from above showing the direction of fire from the ambassadorial suite.

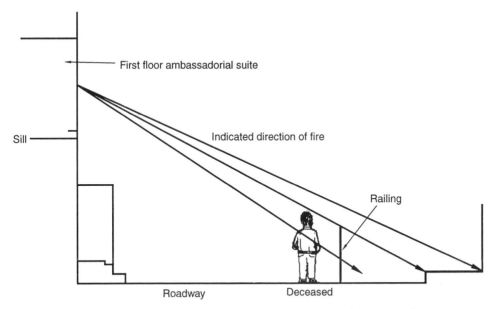

Figure 7.4(b) The side elevation of the scene shown in the previous figure.

Measurement of these, and then comparison with the wound data from the autopsy pointed to the shots having been fired from the first floor at the front of the mission.

When access was finally gained, careful examination of the first floor ambassadorial suite revealed a fired cartridge case of the correct calibre, caught up in the curtains and missed by the perpetrators in their efforts to clear up the scene.

References

Burke T.W. and Rowe W.F. (1992) Bullet ricochet: a comprehensive review. *J. For. Sci.* **37**, 1254–1260.

Copeland A.R. (1984) Accidental death by gunshot wound – fact or fiction. *For. Sci. Int.* **26**, 25–32.

DiMaio V.J.M. (1985) *Gunshot Wounds. Practical Aspects of Firearms, Ballistics and Forensic Techniques*. Elsevier, New York.

DiMaio V.J.M., Dana S.E., Taylor W.E. and Ondrusek J. (1987) Use of scanning electron microscope and energy dispersive X-ray analysis (SEM-EDXA) in identification of foreign material on bullets. *J. For. Sci.* **32**, 38–47.

Dix J.D., Stout S.D. and Mosley J. (1991) Bones, blood, pellets, glass, and no body. *J. For. Sci.* **36**, 949–952.

Gerdin B. (1980) A case of disguised suicide. *For. Sci. Int.* **16**, 29–34.

Haag L.C. (1975) Bullet ricochet: an empirical study and a device for measuring ricochet angle. *AFTE J.* **7**, 44–51.

Janssen D.W. and Levine R.T. (1982) Bullet ricochet from automobile ceilings. *J. For. Sci.* **27**, 209–212.

Jordan G.E., Bratton D.D., Donahue H.C.H. and Rowe W.F. (1988) Bullet ricochet from gypsum wallboard. *J. For. Sci.* **33**, 1477–1482.

Mitosinka G.T. (1971) Technique for determining and illustrating the trajectory of bullets. *J. For. Sci. Soc.* **11**, 55–61.

Murphy G.K. (1989) Suicide by gunshot while driving an automobile. *Am. J. For. Med. Pathol.* **10**, 285–288.

Nennstiel R. (1985) Accuracy in determining long-range firing position of gunman. *AFTE J.* **17**, 47–54.

Reay D.T., Haglund W.D. and Bonnell H.J. (1986) Wah Mee massacre. *Am. J. For. Med. Pathol.* **7**, 330–336.

Roberts J. and Hanby J. (1985) Reconstuction of a shooting to prove/disprove trajectory. *AFTE J.* **17**, 53–55.

CHAPTER 8

Scene type: combustion and explosion deaths

Fires

INTRODUCTION

Owing to increased public awareness of the hazards posed by fire, and the greater attention being paid to fire precautions, the total number of fire deaths in the United Kingdom has fallen over the last decade. Approximately 800 people still die in fires every year (Home Office, 1993). Although 70 per cent of these deaths occur in the home as a result of accidents, nearly 10 per cent of the fires are deliberately started and are likely to be the subject of a detailed police investigation. It may not be immediately apparent from the circumstances surrounding the incident whether a serious crime has in fact taken place. It is therefore essential that arrangements are made for the cause of all fatal fires to be thoroughly investigated. Indeed, the question of suicide, homicide or accident may only be resolved by a combination of scene examination, post-mortem investigation and toxicological analysis. It is advisable that every fatal fire is treated as a suspicious death until the cause of the fire has been established. The examination and removal of the body must proceed upon the assumption that the forensic evidence to support a criminal prosecution may need to be preserved, identified and recovered.

In 1985 the Home Office published a set of guidelines for the police and fire services covering the procedures to be adopted in the event of a fatal fire occurring. These were re-issued in 1992 with some amendments (Home Office, 1985, 1992) and aim to encourage a multi-agency approach to scene investigation, stressing the need for close co-operation between all the parties involved. As a result of this initiative, in many parts of the United Kingdom, special arson investigation teams comprising representatives of the fire brigade, police officers and scenes of crime examiners have been set up to deal with fatal fires and other incidents (Woodward, 1985). Such teams include forensic scientists, pathologists and forensic medical examiners as the circumstances and local arrangements warrant. A multidisciplinary approach to fire investigation is essential; the skills involved in establishing the cause of a fire are not easily come by. Expertise in fire investigation is based upon the accumulation of extensive practical experience in the field and a sound knowledge of fire science. The non-practitioner should not be tempted into carrying out an investigation into the cause of any fire if a better qualified person is available.

SCENE ASSESSMENT AND PRESERVATION

The very first consideration at any fire scene, once the fire has been put out, should be for the safety of those persons who will be responsible for recovering the body and investigating the cause of the fire. The Health and Safety at Work, etc., Act 1974 is applicable to all those who attend fire scenes, and requires them to take any reasonably practicable steps to ensure their own safety and the safety of others while they are working on the site.

Fire-damaged buildings pose certain hazards that are not normally encountered at other scenes of crime. A fire can destroy the structural integrity of a building, leaving floors weakened, and walls and ceilings unsupported. As a result, parts of the building will be prone to failure, if they are disturbed by post-fire settlement or by the weight of a person walking on them. Before entering the premises, an assessment of structure safety should be made; cracked or leaning walls or wooden floors, which have been severely damaged from below, should be treated with caution as they could fail without warning. The same is true of stonework, which may crack internally due to thermal stresses generated during the fire, and then break up and collapse as it cools and contracts. In premises where structural collapse has already occurred, there may be loose masonry and timbers overhead, and broken glass, protruding nails and other sharp objects in the debris underfoot. It is essential that anyone entering the premises be protected from these hazards. Boots with reinforced insoles and ankle protection, sturdy gloves, a helmet and overalls should be regarded as part of the normal equipment for use when visiting any fire scene. In cold conditions, protective clothing should include garments chosen for warmth, as prolonged exposure to low temperatures will inevitably lead to physical and mental impairment. In some circumstances, the wearing of face masks or respirators may also be appropriate, where hazardous or irritating dusts or vapours are present. Such respirators are no protection against asphyxiants and some toxic gases, so the premises should be thoroughly ventilated before work begins (normally this would be part of routine fire-fighting procedures). In all instances, when assessing the safety of fire scenes a simple rule should be followed: if there is any doubt about the safety of a course of action, then it should be avoided.

With large buildings, or those that incorporate unusual materials or methods of construction, it is advisable that a structural engineer be called to assess the site before work begins. If the hazard extends to areas normally accessible to the general public, then the local borough surveyor or building safety officer may insist upon remedial work being carried out before scene investigation begins. Specialist advice should be sought after fires in industrial premises where there may be hazards associated with the processes that are carried out on site. Some older industrial buildings may also contain asbestos insulation, which can be released during a fire. The concentration of asbestos fibres in the atmosphere can be monitored with special equipment and, if it is above recommended safety levels (Health and Safety Executive, 1984), then advice should be taken from a qualified source such as an environmental health officer, before entering the building. Hazards arising from the nature of the building's occupancy may not simply be confined to industrial premises. Squats and semi-derelict houses are frequently used by vagrants and drug addicts, and such premises may contain biohazards such as used syringes and needles. Extreme care should be exercised when moving bodies and clearing debris in such buildings; equipment should be disinfected if it has come into contact with contaminated material.

Once the safety of persons working at the scene has been assured, then efforts should be made to preserve evidence from further damage. A perimeter must be established that encompasses all the areas of potential interest and access to that part of the site should be carefully controlled. If the presence of a flammable liquid is suspected, then particular care must be taken to protect those areas where it might have been distributed, since the pattern of distribution within the premises may be the only evidence that allows the investigator to distinguish between internal and external attack. Analytical techniques currently used by forensic science laboratories are sufficiently sensitive that even the small quantities of flammable liquid accidentally transferred on the shoes of a person walking through the premises could be recovered and misinterpreted.

EXAMINATION OF THE BODY

After the safety and security of the premises have been assured, the forensic medical examiner can certify death. Access to the body may be difficult if the floor it is resting on has been weakened, but ladders and scaffold boards can be laid across remaining sturdy joists to provide a stable platform from which to work. If the internal stairs have collapsed, then ladders may also need to be stepped from outside the building to the windows of the room where the victim is lying. Death should be certified with the minimum of disturbance to the body and clothing. The victim should then be left *in situ* for the scene examination; there is a considerable amount of evidence to be gained from the position and condition of the body, all of which can be lost if it is moved prematurely.

Once the initial photographs and sketches of the body have been made, any loose fallen debris can be removed and the exposed, surfaces can be rephotographed and examined for evidence of non-accidental injury or signs of loose personal effects. The body should then be lifted, or rolled over on to a plastic sheet or body bag. Heavy-duty gloves should be worn to move the body as the loose debris present may contain sharp objects and there will nearly always be the risk of body-fluid contamination when handling fire victims. Disposable latex gloves or washing-up gloves do not provide adequate protection at fire scenes but, if no better alternative is available then at least two pairs should always be worn.

The contact surfaces of the body and the material it is resting on should be photographed and, if necessary, notes should be made of the condition of the clothing and skin. If the victim has been lying *in situ* for most of the fire then protected areas where the clothing and, for example, floor coverings have been in contact, will be apparent. If on the other hand the fire started on the victim's clothing, and collapse occurred as a result of burns, then it is likely that the fabrics trapped between the body and the floor will show signs of burning or melting. If the fire appears to have been confined to the victim's clothing then the distribution of the damage is of great importance. Accidental ignition of clothing can occur for a number of reasons but the point of ignition is very much dependent upon the ignition source. Severe burns to one sleeve or arm, and the destruction of upper portions of the clothing on that side of the body may indicate contact with an open flame, such as a lit gas hob, while reaching across it (Figure 8.1).

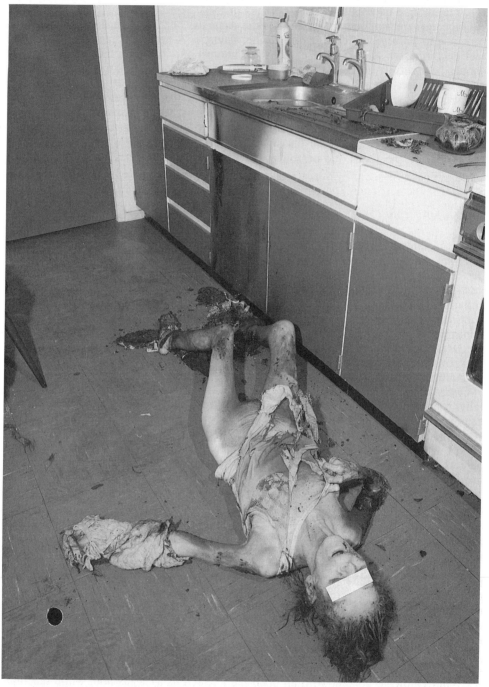

Figure 8.1 An elderly female shown lying on her kitchen floor near her cooker. She had reached over with her right hand, making contact with an open flame of a lit gas hob. Note that the clothing covering her right arm and upper part of her body on that side have burnt away. The victim collapsed while attempting to put herself out at the sink.

A fire originating in the lap area is more likely, however, to be due to a burning item being dropped there, possibly as the result of an accident with smoking materials. In accidents of this type, the victim may well move away from the place where his or her clothing caught fire, and go to a sink or basin in order to try to put the flames out or cool the burns. This movement can leave a trail of burnt fabric through the premises and, if the victim has collapsed by a sink, there may be fragments of burnt clothing in the drain. The context in which the victim is found will often provide evidence of a sequence of events from which the location of the ignition source can be deduced. In most cases, extensive burning to the clothing will result in the rapid collapse of the victim due to shock. On rare occasions, the victim may behave with paradoxical normality before collapse; even when suffering from serious injuries, people have changed out of burnt clothing and cleaned up the remains for disposal. Such peculiar behaviour has led to flame burns being wrongly attributed to scalding on the grounds that there was no sign of a fire at the scene and the victim's clothing was intact when inspected during post-mortem. A search of waste bins in the premises is advisable in these circumstances as this will often reveal the remnants of the clothing the victim was actually wearing at the time of the fire.

In cases where the victim has not sustained burns but has collapsed at a point remote from the fire, the body and its surroundings will have been affected only by smoke spread. The pattern of smoke deposits will reveal whether the body has been moved, a distinct possibility when firemen search smoke-filled rooms. If the victim has been overcome by smoke, then the position and orientation of the body, together with the items around it, may provide evidence that the victim was aware of the fire and perhaps trying to extinguish it or escape. Wet towels, pans, bowls and kettles have all been found beside victims who have collapsed while attempting to fight fires.

CONCEALED HOMICIDE

Disposal of a murder victim by burning is not at all uncommon and the investigators should be on their guard at all times when investigating a fatal fire. Careful post-mortem and scene investigation, followed by toxicological analysis, especially to ascertain the presence and level of carboxyhaemoglobin saturation in blood, will enable the correct assessment to be made.

It is frequently the case that a substantial portion of the body is severely burnt and most external signs of violence may have been destroyed. However, internal examination is much more helpful because, even with badly burnt bodies internal organs are present and, even though sometimes altered by heat, an assessment of any injuries is easier.

Remnants of clothing and documents at the scene must be treated with great care because of their fragility due to heat destruction and, furthermore, they may have been separated from the body (burnt off), although lying adjacent to it. Their position should be carefully documented prior to collection.

CASE 8.1
A young woman was found dead in her bedroom. Her 4-year-old daughter was found alive in another upstairs room and was able to give the police a brief story about 'one of the daddies lighting mummy with matches'. Her mother was a prostitute and had frequent clients calling round. The seat of the fire was established as occurring on the side of her bed nearest her right hand (Figure 8.2(a)). The murderer had deliberately

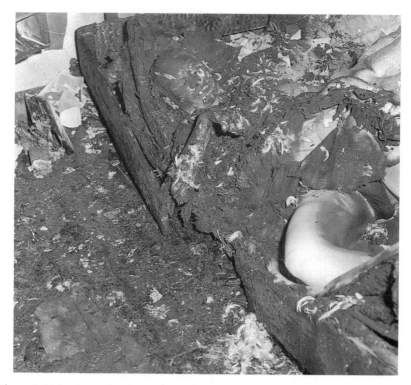

Figure 8.2(a)   A murder victim shown lying on bed. She had been set alight after she had been strangled. The seat of fire is on the side of her bed nearest to her right hand.

set fire to that side of her bed in order to deceive the investigators into thinking that she had dropped a lighted cigarette whilst in bed. On examination of the body, after cleaning and extending her neck, it became obvious that she had been strangled with a ligature (Figure 8.2(b)). She had no soot in her airways and there was no carboxyhaemoglobin found in her blood.

ESTABLISHING THE CAUSE OF THE FIRE

Once the body has been removed, the scene examination proper can be carried out. Fire spread creates certain characteristic patterns of damage within a building. Smoke and hot gases, being less dense than the cooler air present before a fire, will tend to rise in a room and then spread outwards beneath the ceiling. A hot gas layer will accumulate at high level within the compartment in which the fire is burning, then spill through the tops of doorways and other openings into adjacent areas. If the buoyant fire gases reach a vertical shaft, such as a stairwell, then they will rise up it rather than spread outwards at a lower level (this is referred to as the 'chimney effect'). In order to replace the hot gases escaping from the area of origin, cold air will be drawn in through the lower parts of any openings, thus providing the oxygen needed to sustain the fire.

After the fire has been extinguished an inspection may reveal that many of the rooms

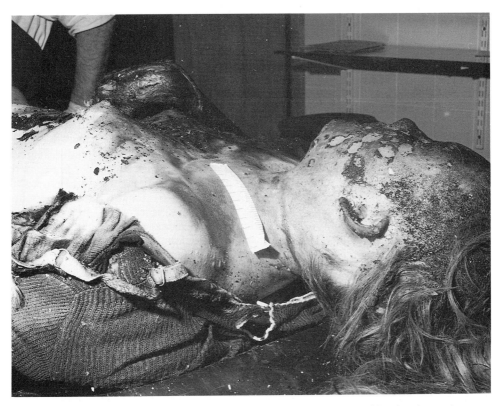

Figure 8.2(b) A ligature mark on the victim's neck is clearly visible after the neck was cleaned and extended slightly in the mortuary.

in the building are only burnt or smoke-stained at high level and can therefore be classified as areas affected only by fire spread. Elimination of these rooms should leave only a relatively small number of areas that will need to be examined in detail. Once the area of interest has been defined it should be photographed before anything is moved; two photographs from diagonally opposite corners of a room will normally cover the entire floor and the contents satisfactorily.

The debris in the room can then be cleared in order to afford a better view of the damage to the structure and contents. The clearance must be carried out with care so that fragile materials are retained *in situ* or recovered for later replacement. The lowest layer of debris should also be smelt in case flammable liquid residues are present. Portable hydrocarbon vapour detectors are available and are often used by the fire brigade to survey the scene for traces of fire accelerants such as petrol or kerosene. Such instruments, which are generally referred to as 'sniffers', must be used with care as they are broad-spectrum devices and not specifically detectors of accelerants, and the combustion of the synthetic materials, which are used to make furniture and carpets, produces hydrocarbon pyrolysis products that give false positive readings. If the presence of a flammable liquid is suspected, then a sample of the material into which the liquid has soaked should be taken for analysis. Debris samples should be secured in non-permeable packaging; nylon bags are suitable for hydrocarbon-based liquids such as petrol, paraffin, white spirit or diesel fuel, but polar liquids such as alcohols and certain types of thinners must be placed in glass jars or metal containers as nylon is permeable to polar compounds. The excavation of loose fallen debris is essential in order to reveal the state of the original contents and permit the reconstruction of items that were present at the time of the fire. These can then be positioned using marks left on the walls and floor where areas have been protected from damage.

After reconstruction, the pattern of fire damage at the scene can be assessed and the likely area of origin of the fire established. The seat or seats of the fire will normally be identifiable as the lowest points of burning in the areas exhibiting the greatest degree of fire damage. Only after the area of origin has been found can potential ignition sources be identified by establishing what was actually present in the area when the fire started. It is not sufficient to identify a source of ignition within the premises and assume that this was the cause of the fire; viable sources such as gas fires and electric heaters are common, but, if these appliances are not within the area of origin, then they cannot have started the fire. Certain types of ignition source produce characteristic patterns of damage, which, if not obscured by the subsequent development of the fire, will indicate how the fire started.

Smouldering fires initiated by cigarettes give rise to severe localised charring before they reach the stage where flames are produced. The presence of such an area of intense damage, for example, on foam-padded furniture may point towards smouldering smoking materials as the source of ignition. In contrast, widespread but very evenly distributed damage could be the result of a fire that has been flaming from the start.

Many accidental fatal fires result from the abuse or misuse of heaters or cooking appliances, the controls of which should be inspected to determine whether they were on or off at the time. The condition of such appliances should be carefully assessed. Inspection may reveal burnt or melted materials adhering to heating elements or safety grilles. Cooking accidents involving the boil-over of deep friers will leave a layer of fat or oil on the hob, and the pan itself may still be present, if it has not been moved either by the victim or during fire fighting. A more detailed discussion of the methods used to establish the precise cause of a fire are beyond the scope of this book and are covered elsewhere (DeHaan, 1983; Cooke and Ide, 1985).

Owing to the preponderance of accidental fatal fires, the habits and activities of the victim may be of considerable importance when looking for a cause of the fire. A combination of elevated blood alcohol levels and smoking is frequently reported at inquest, and evidence of the victim's drinking habits may be readily apparent. Advanced age, infirmity, poor living conditions, and social or religious customs can all be associated with enhanced fire risk. There is a possibility that the fatal fire being investigated is the culmination of a series of minor incidents; evidence of previous fires may be apparent upon examining the premises or there may be a history of accidents. Sources of information on the victim's lifestyle include relatives, friends, neighbours and, in the case of the elderly or disabled, the social services. When considering information obtained from these sources, it must be borne in mind that they may not be in possession of the true facts; fire victims are known to have successfully concealed the fact that they smoked, even from close relatives. When there is a conflict between witness information and the facts established at the scene by examination, the latter should be regarded as the more reliable evidence.

'SPONTANEOUS' HUMAN COMBUSTION

In some fires, the body of the victim may display exceptionally severe localised damage, while materials in the immediate vicinity appear to be unaffected. Often the victim's torso is partly or completely consumed and large bones reduced to a crumbly grey ash. Many observers of this phenomenon, in trying to reconcile the conditions they know are required to cremate a body with those which must have been present at the scene, explain the damage in terms of a supernatural 'fire from within'. Spontaneous human combustion (SHC) is the popular term for such fires and it has also been used as an explanation for fatal fires where no ignition source has been found. The classic case histories of SHC originated in the nineteenth century, and often revolved around a victim who would consume large quantities of spirits and then retire for the night. Later the victim would either be seen burning or found partly burnt away with no apparent cause. With the prevalence of open fires and candles in those times, it is hardly surprising that an intoxicated person might suffer an accident. However, nineteenth century fascination with the supernatural, coupled with influential fictional accounts from authors of the time, demanded a less prosaic explanation for such incidents. For similar reasons, SHC has its supporters even to the present day despite scientific scepticism (Adelson, 1981; Nickell and Fischer, 1984).

Quoted instances of SHC where there is severe damage to the body, rely upon a mistaken attempt to draw an analogy between the process of cremation and the conditions it is claimed must be present for a fire completely to destroy flesh and bone. Cremation involves the destruction of a body using a furnace fitted with gas burners operating at high temperatures, conditions which are intended to make the process as quick and efficient as possible (Petty, 1978). Most domestic fires resulting in the partial or complete destruction of a body are, however, neither quick nor particularly efficient but, given enough time, even a relatively small flame is capable of causing massive damage. The essential requirement is that the fire around the body is provided with a source of fuel, which will sustain it for the time needed to burn away the flesh and calcine the exposed bone. In many instances the fuel is supplied by the body itself in the form of liquefied fat rendered out from the tissues as they are heated (Figure 8.3). Such fires do tend to be more common with victims who are obese as they can provide a greater quantity of fat to fuel the fire, allowing it to burn for longer. If there is an absorbent material nearby, which is capable of acting as a wick, such as the victim's clothing, then the fat will burn as if in an oil lamp, and the process of rendering and tissue destruction will continue, sometimes leaving only the extremities around a hole in the floor.

In the case described by Gee (1965), however, the deceased was a slim elderly female who had collapsed near an open fire. It was thought that her head had been ignited first by the fire. The prolonged combustibility confined to the deceased was thought to be due to the body being in the draught from the chimney, thus preventing the spread of flames from the lighted fire to other parts of the room. Fires in such circumstances tend to leave very greasy smoke deposits within the premises but may not spread beyond the immediate vicinity of the body, if there are no readily combustible items nearby.

Small fires involving the almost complete destruction of the victim's body are rare. They appear to be very sensitive to ambient conditions and are entirely dependent upon the fire not being discovered for a considerable period of time. This very rarity has been regarded as a reason for suggesting an unnatural origin for the fire. Certain otherwise unremarkable fires are also attributed to SHC on the grounds that there was no

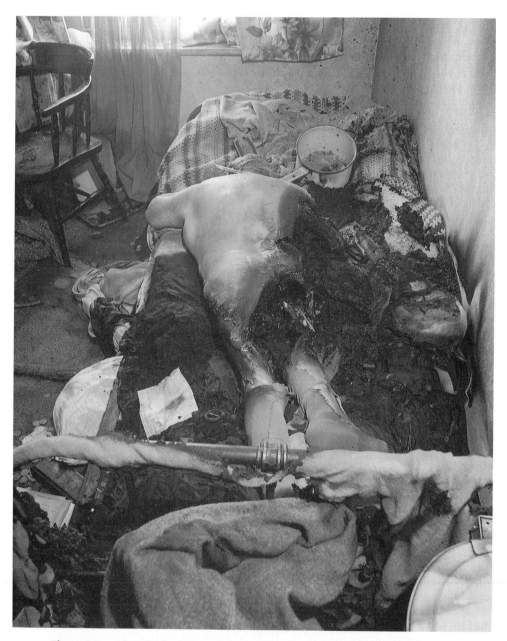

Figure 8.3 A homicide victim in which there has been prolonged and localised post-mortem burning, which has severed her right leg. On her left side are seen a collection of blisters containing liquefied body fat.

apparent ignition source at the scene. It is possible that most, if not all of these incidents have been complicated by the actions of the victim who may have moved away from, turned off or disconnected the ignition source before collapse occurred. It is also worth bearing in mind that young witnesses to the reportedly sourceless ignition of clothing may be reluctant to admit that they had been playing with lighters or matches at the time.

MULTIPLE FATALITIES AND MAJOR DISASTERS

Scenes where there has been a major loss of life will always pose problems for those trying to establish the identity of victims. Fires are no exception to this rule; indeed, the problem of identity is exacerbated by the destruction of clothing and personal effects, and, in addition, severe damage to the body itself may render it impossible or inadvisable for relatives to identify it. Appropriate steps should be taken to record all relevant information and preserve materials associated with the bodies as they are recovered in order to facilitate the process of identification.

The large-scale nature of such incidents inevitably means that victim recovery is a team effort, often involving the use of persons with limited training in forensic recovery methods. Adequate supervision of site teams is essential from the start as it is in the early stages of scene work that mistakes are often made.

The removal of the victims before site procedures have been agreed is not advisable; a planned approach is likely to yield the maximum amount of useful information. During the control phase of a major incident, fire services should be encouraged to leave bodies *in situ* unless they are impeding fire fighting or rescue operations. Experiences at Denmark Place in London, Bradford City football ground and King's Cross station, highlight the importance of preserving bodies and associated materials from the moment they are found.

One person on the site team should be given the responsibility for ensuring that the position of each body is noted and that identification evidence is recovered intact. He or she should also supervise the recovery teams as they remove the body and associated materials.

As each body is uncovered it should be given a unique identifying number or letter, which should be clearly displayed in the photographs. This identifier should also be marked with indelible ink on a waterproof label, which can be firmly attached to the body, not the bag or coffin it is removed in. The debris in the area surrounding the body should be searched before it is moved and any personal effects in the immediate vicinity should be recovered, labelled appropriately, then sealed inside the body bag and sent with the body to the casualty reception point. Only at the reception point should personal effects be sorted and examined. Any attempt to separate out such items at the fire ground will only lead to confusion and possibly to an incorrect identification (the dire effects of the latter on the relatives of a victim should be all the justification required for these procedures).

Before the body itself is lifted, any severely burnt or fragile extremities such as the hands, head and feet should be covered with polythene bags to retain jewellery, clothing and bone remnants. If the flesh on the face has been lost, then it is likely that the front teeth will be burnt. A layer of cling film over the mouth will prevent the teeth from breaking up during removal and preserve them for dental identification if it proves necessary.

The investigation of fatal explosions

SITUATIONS IN WHICH EXPLOSIONS MAY OCCUR

Scenes of explosions can be divided into three categories:

1. Those where high explosives have been used.
2. Those involving dispersed phase explosives.
3. Those which have been damaged by mechanical explosions.

Most of the procedures for recovering the body and investigating such incidents are the same as for any other sudden death, with the proviso that in industrial premises or at large-scale incidents the Health and Safety Executive or a nominated body such as British Gas may have a statutory duty to investigate the cause.

Incidents arising from the use of *high explosives* are usually related to terrorist offences. At scenes where a high-explosive device has operated, the only action to be taken by other services should be to contain and secure the scene pending the arrival of the proper authorities. No entry or search should be conducted as there is a possibility that further devices or booby-traps could be present.

Dispersed phase explosions are those which have been caused by gas, flammable vapours or combustible dusts.

Mechanical explosions arise from the sudden release of pressure when a sealed container such as a gas cylinder ruptures.

In industrial concerns, explosions may arise from such items as compressed air tanks, equipment using steam under pressure, furnaces, boilers, finely pulverised coal dust in mine shafts, flour dust in mills and granaries, or pulverised sawdust. In the industrial situation, safety-directed engineering devices are often built into such potentially explosive loci and will ensure that the effects of any such explosions are limited and localised, and loss of life and casualties are often on a small scale.

In the domestic situation, the ignition of vapours of flammable substances, e.g., gasoline, and the escape of gases, e.g., butane cylinders and domestic 'natural gas' supplies, may also cause very serious explosions; a mixture of 'natural gas' in a one in ten mixture with air in a confined space can be readily ignited by a spark from an electrical appliance.

Meteorological phenomena such as lightning strikes may also produce explosions.

EFFECTS OF AN EXPLOSION

It is essential for the correct interpretation of the scene to understand the effects of an explosion, which may be summarised as follows:

1. A direct blast force, i.e., pressure or mechanical waves are generated, lasting a few milliseconds, and moving out concentrically from the explosion epicentre, followed by a negative pressure suction-type wave. The semivacuum formed by the initial blast wave is refilled with air rushing back in.
2. Hot gases are generated which may cause fires in the vicinity and flash burns in victims.
3. There is fragmentation of components of the explosive device and other items in the vicinity, causing missile injuries in victims. Some terrorist devices are packed with metal nails and similar objects.

4. There is frequently destruction of buildings or other nearby structures causing injuries to victims, particularly from falling masonary.

The severity of an explosion can vary considerably and the damage may range from the loss of a few window panes to the complete destruction of a multistorey structure. Most dispersed-phase explosions are deflagrations – extremely rapid fires – and the damage they cause is due to the pressure rise induced in the building when large amounts of hot combustion gases are produced. This pressure rise is progressively relieved by the failure of the weakest components of the structure until sufficient venting has occurred, at which point no more structural damage other than collapse will take place. Similar structural damage is caused by mechanical explosions, but the cylinder or other container may also be propelled a considerable distance when its pressurised contents are released.

Owing to the likelihood of structural damage, the same care should be exercised at scenes of explosions as at fires and the premises should be assessed for safety before work begins. Body recovery will be made more difficult if large amounts of collapsed masonry have to be removed, and it may be necessary to organise site teams and obtain mechanical assistance to remove heavy objects. At large explosions, bodies as well as survivors are likely to be uncovered during rescue work, and it is advisable that any recovery and identification procedures developed for major incidents be implemented as part of the rescue services operations.

FINDINGS IN BODIES

The findings in bodies, which are discovered in the vicinity of the explosion, are extremely variable and to a major extent depend on the physical siting of the victim in relation to the seat of the explosion and the severity of the blast.

As a general rule, and particularly when dealing with multiple deaths, many parts of bodies can be expected to be strewn over a very wide area. In a recent case involving a terrorist bombing of an army barracks, the disrupted remains of the person nearest to the explosive device were found further away than those of his other fatally injured colleagues.

The type, extent and distribution of injuries, together with associated debris, either on the surface or within the body, will assist the scene investigators in locating the position of each person at the moment the explosion took place. Bodies within 1 or 2 metres of the explosion will frequently be severely disrupted. Injuries in bodies, which are lying over 2 metres from the explosion, show a picture consisting of punctate and speckled lacerations and abrasions, often circular and oval bruises, which are scattered throughout the exposed parts of the body. Their concentration on the surface of the body is variable but may be very extensive. These are caused by debris and shrapnel from the blast coming into forceful contact with the skin to produce wounding and may even become embedded in the tissues, or penetrate deeply into muscle compartments and body cavities. For a detailed description of such injuries the reader may wish to consult the work of Marshall (1976, 1978, 1988).

Frequently, flying debris from the centre of an explosion cause wounding, which has an orientation in the direction of the blast. This is also assisted by the position of any flash burns that are present. Hair may also have a 'swept back' appearance where the deceased was facing the blast.

Although not strictly part of the scene investigation, radiography (an essential procedure to be carried out in each case prior to autopsy), may enable identification of foreign bodies, which have come from an explosive device, as well as assist in identification of the body.

Furthermore it should be appreciated that, especially when dealing with a perpetrator who was carrying an explosive device, and has died as a result of its accidental or deliberate detonation, the distribution of injuries and fragments found in the deceased, his or her position at the scene, as well as identification of his or her remains, will enable an accurate assessment to be made of his or her role in the incident.

Bodies found away from the immediate area where the explosion has occurred will frequently have suffered mechanical injuries due to falling masonry from the collapse of a building.

Dispersed-phase explosions do not produce the high-velocity penetration wounds typical of high explosives but, if the victim was within the burning gas or vapour then flash-burns will be present on the body and clothing.

INVESTIGATING THE CAUSE OF THE EXPLOSION

Investigating the cause of a major explosion is very time consuming as it requires the recovery and inspection of much of the contents of the structure. With minor explosions, it may be possible to identify the origin by plotting a displacement diagram showing direction of movement of walls, doors and windows during the incident. The diagram may indicate a single room of origin, which can then be excavated and inspected in order to establish whether a dispersed-phase or a mechanical explosion has occurred. Dispersed-phase explosions, involving as they do the combustion of a fuel/air mixture, leave evidence of heat damage from the passage of the flame front through the premises. Mechanical explosions are not always caused by a combustion-related process, although most arise from the rupture of a sealed container, which has been heated in a fire. Distinguishing between the two is possible if it can be established whether there was a fire within the premises before the explosion occurred, or whether there were sealed or pressurised gas or water systems present.

The most common fuels encountered in dispersed-phase explosions are methane (natural gas from the mains), propane (Calor gas), butane (camping gas) and the vapours from volatile flammable liquids such as petrol. Of these, only methane is less dense than air in the vapour phase and, as a result, it tends to accumulate in a layer above the point of release, while propane, butane and petrol vapour will all form layers at low level unless disturbed by draughts. When the gas or vapour is ignited this stratification leads to an uneven pattern of burning or scorching of exposed surfaces, which can aid the identification of the explosive material. This burning is very superficial and should not be confused with the damage caused by a fire after the explosion or flaring from a broken gas supply pipe. If the presence of a vapour or gas denser than air is indicated, then a search must be made for flammable liquid residues or cylinders. Most gas explosions are the result of accidental release, but appliances and pipework should be examined for evidence of tampering or attempts to bypass the meter. The presence of flammable liquid should be regarded as a cause for suspicion unless there is good reason for such material to be present. Containers in the vicinity of the body may indicate that the victim was caught in a vapour explosion after having distributed a flammable liquid around the premises.

Essentially, the main aims of the forensic scientist in such instances are:

1. To detect any residual undetonated explosive residues by collecting appropriate samples often embedded in soft porous materials, such as wood, soil or insulating materials, and on the surface of metallic objects.
2. To collect as much information as possible about the features and construction of the explosive device.

For a detailed treatment of explosion investigation techniques, outside the scope of this book, the reader is referred to Harris (1983) and Yallop (1980).

References

Adelson L. (1981) Spontaneous human combustion and preternatural combustibility. *Fire Arson Invest.* **31**, 38–55.
Cooke R.A. and Ide R.H. (1985) *Principles of Fire Investigation.* Institute of Fire Engineers.
DeHaan J.D. (1983) *Kirk's Fire Investigation*, 2nd edn. John Wiley & Sons, New York.
Gee D.J. (1965) A case of 'spontaneous combustion'. *Med. Sci. Law* **5**, 37–38.
Harris R.J. (1983) The investigation and control of gas explosions. In *Buildings and Heating Plant*, pp.121–138. E. & F.N. Spon Ltd, London.
Health and Safety Executive (1984) *Asbestos – Control Limits. Measurement of Airborne Dust Concentrations and the Assessment of Control Measures.* Environmental Series Guidance Note EH1O. HMSO, London.
Home Office Circular 71/1985. *The Investigation of Fires of Doubtful Origin.* Home Office, London.
Home Office Circular 106/1992. *The Investigation of Fires of Doubtful Origin.* Home Office, London.
Marshall T.K. (1976) Death from explosive devices. *Med. Sci. Law* **16**, 235–239.
Marshall T.K. (1978) The investigation of bombings. In Wecht C. (ed.) *Legal Medicine Annual*, pp. 37–59. Appleton Century Crofts, New York.
Marshall T.K. (1988) A pathologist's view of terrorist violence. *For. Sci. Int.* **36**, 57–67.
Nickell J. and Fischer J.F. (1984) Spontaneous human combustion. *Fire Arson Invest.* **34**, 4–11.
Petty C.S. (1978) Fire death identification and pathology. *Fire Arson Invest.* **28**, 36.
Summary Fire Statistics, United Kingdom 1992 (1993) Home Office Statistical Bulletin 28/93. Home Office, London.
Woodward E.H. (1985) Investigation of arson. The Cleveland Experiment. *Police J.* **2**, 111–117.
Yallop H.J. (1980) *Explosion Investigation.* The Forensic Science Society and Scottish Academic Press, Harrogate and Edinburgh.

CHAPTER 9

Scene type: deaths of children

The investigation of suspicious deaths involving children is frequently one of the most problematic areas in forensic investigation. The scenario frequently involves a young child who has suffered multiple episodes of trauma at the hands of its custodians, be they parents, guardians or others; in only a very few cases, is the person responsible a complete stranger.

Examination of the scene in such cases is necessary, particularly to ascertain whether injuries are compatible with being caused by various items or surfaces within that environment in the manner described by the custodians.

Suspected child abuse cases

When a child is found dead, usually in a domestic environment or dies later in hospital, the carers are questioned closely to elicit the explanation for any injuries. The investigators, including the pathologist, then have the task of assessing the credibility of any accounts given. Frequently such an assessment cannot be made without a thorough examination of the child's environment, where the injuries were allegedly caused. In view of the fact that most injured children are taken to hospital and are either brought in dead or die at a later time, the scene is, of necessity, examined retrospectively in the vast majority of cases. In actual fact, scene examination and reconstruction of events, armed with a full knowledge of the extent of the injuries and possibly accounts by carers as to how injuries were caused, is much more preferable than examining the scene before the autopsy has been completed. It has to be accepted, however, that, because of the absence of a body from the scene in many cases, the scene examination in some instances is unfortunately either neglected or not considered as thoroughly as is necessary (Wagner, 1986).

The most common cause of death in the battered child syndome involves some form of blunt head injury for which various explanations may be forthcoming from the suspects. Indeed, it is not uncommon for a suspect to attempt to explain a severe head injury or an injury to some other part of the body, by some accidental means. It is vital therefore to interpret such injuries in the light of explanations offered, in conjuction

Table 9.1 Explanations offered by parents/guardians in 29 cases of the battered child syndrome (Cameron et al., 1966).

No.	Original story	Probable truth
1	Fell from pram and caught ear on handle.	Three blows on face and then bounced on floor.
2	Fell and caught stomach against door.	Mother kicked him in stomach.
3	Fell downstairs; fell against stove and table. Fell off fence, off chair. Stomach ache – something he drank.	Five blows, kicking him and striking with broom handle (father). Struck with fist and shoe and hitting stomach (mother).
4	Fell off settee and hit head against table.	Blow with hand behind left ear.
5	Tripped whilst carrying baby.	Threw him to the floor.
6	Fell and hit head on grate.	Head injury and belt marks and bruises on back and legs. Denied responsibility.
7	'Must have fallen out of pram'.	Crushed against bannister and thrown downstairs.
8	Fell downstairs whilst carrying child.	Thrown downstairs.
9	Child 'kept coming out in bruises'.	Scratched abdomen with engagement ring and multiple blows.
10	Fell downstairs with baby.	Threw baby downstairs – injury to head.
11	Toppled backwards whilst sitting on grass.	Blows on face and head.
12	Older brother fell over.	Dropped on floor.
13	Fell off bed on to face.	Father lost temper after being on night shift.
14	Fall from pram.	Kicked in stomach.
15	Fall from table to floor while left alone.	Father lost temper and threw child into chair with wooden arms, twice.
16	Pyloric stenosis and hiatus hernia. Fell against door.	Father lost temper and hit child with hand hurling him against the edge of the sink.
17	Mother fell downstairs and dropped baby.	Threw baby downstairs on concrete floor.
18	Fell off bed, pulled furniture on himself.	Dropped child on head.
19	Fell out of pram.	Dragged by scruff of neck, gripped by ankles, with multiple fractures.
20	Fell downstairs 3 days prior to death.	Lost temper and hit child. Died suddenly.
21	Died after feed; father tried to save it falling from knee.	Admitted hitting child with hand.
22	Dropped baby on floor.	Repeated blows with open hand.
23	Father fell downstairs while carrying child – arm caught between bannisters.	Blows administered by step-father. Resuscitation.
24	Mother admitted ill-treatment and had resorted to force feeding.	As admitted.
25	Fell off table and vomited.	Admitted hitting child then tried to gas herself.
26	Must have strayed too near the fire.	Father held child against the electric fire. Multiple blows.
27	Denied all knowledge initially.	Father lost temper, slapped face, threw into carry-cot, slapped face again. Repeated blows.
28	None given.	Repeated blows.
29	Spilt water over herself.	Persistent ill-treatment with multiple blows.

with the scene. Head injuries in particular, should be evaluated, for example, with respect to distance through which the child has reportedly fallen, to assess whether or not accounts given by the accused are consistent with the injuries found. In many cases such accounts are either 'half truths' or entirely incompatible with the trauma found. Cameron et al. (1966) detailed the original story given, with the eventual truthful story, in 29 cases (Table 9.1). They found that, in the majority of cases, the explanation offered

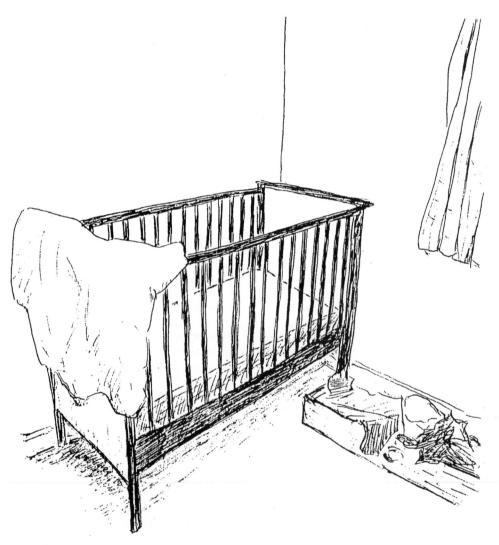

Figure 9.1(a)   A view of a typical cot requiring careful assessment to evaluate any account given where injury is said to have arisen as a result of contact with the sides, for example, or by the child climbing out of it and falling onto the floor. The distance from the top of the cot to the floor should be measured as well as the space between the bars. A general assessment of the cot should also be made to see how stable it is, and, indeed, whether it is broken or faulty in any way.

was one of a simple fall – from cot to floor, pram to ground, against furniture or down a flight of stairs. When the parents or guardians were challenged on the grounds of the inconsistencies between their stories and the injuries seen, they offered further explanations, in some cases suggesting that they were sustained as a result of attempts at resuscitation.

Common aspects of the scene, which the pathologist therefore needs to consider include:

- Heights from the floor of the child's cot and furniture surfaces, such as a chair or a bed, from which a child may have fallen, in conjunction with the type of floor covering.
- Heights of furniture as well as window sills, balcony railings, etc., will also enable the examiner to assess whether or not it was feasible for the child to clamber up or over such structures (Figure 9.1(a) and (b)).
- Assessment type of material and hardness of surface of items of furniture.
- Shape of objects and surfaces, which may match up with injuries found on the child (Figure 9.2).

Burns may have a characteristic pattern, which can be matched, for example, with a radiator grill. Scalding by being held in a bath tub may occasionally be seen. The design of the bath or basin in which the child has received scalds needs to be examined, and measurements taken and related to the burns seen on the child.

CASE 9.1
A 16-month-old infant presented to the casualty department with scalds distributed as shown in Fig 9.3(a). The pattern of scalding clearly indicates that the child had been held in the bath and the hot water tap turned on. Infant's buttocks were pressed against the bottom of the bath and the knees doubled up (Figure 9.3(b)), thus producing the demarcation line between the scalded and the spared area of skin.

It is also essential, as was demonstrated in the following case, to examine the type of water taps, assess the rate of flow of water and the rapidity with which the maximum temperature is reached.

CASE 9.2
A 4-month-old boy was admitted to hospital with partial thickness burns estimated as 65 per cent of body surface area. The mother's explanation for the burns was that she had washed him under a mixer tap in a sink, within a communal kitchen of her lodgings. She was not aware anything was wrong until the child's skin began to peel off in the towel. The mother, according to her sister, was suffering from some form of mental disorder. It was essential for the police to confirm her account by carrying out a thorough scene examination. The pathologist visited the scene accompanied by a scene of crime officer. The sink in the kitchen was found to have a mixer hot and cold water tap. The temperature at its highest was noted to be 58 °C and unbearably hot to an adult hand for longer than one second. The sink was measured and the height of the child also taken into account. The child could not have stood in the sink, but could have been sat with his feet hanging over the edge of the sink. However, the distribution of the burns was more consistent with the child having been directly under the mixer tap. The mother then related that the child had been seated in the bath, which was in the adjoining room, with the head just below the tap, which was then turned on. This explanation appeared to be more compatible with the injuries. An examination of the multipoint water heater, which

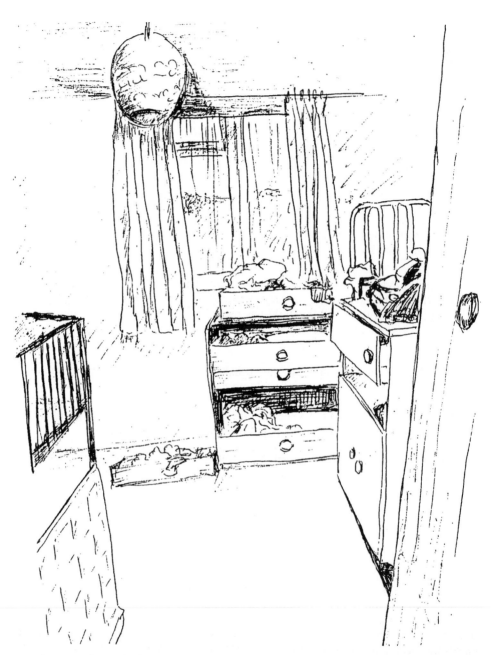

Figure 9.1(b) A further view of the same room and cot as in the previous figure. The position of the window and whether or not it is locked should be ascertained. An assessment should be made of whether or not a child, given its age, could have climbed up the furniture and opened the window. The furniture should be examined in order to assess its relevance to injury causation. The type of flooring and its relative hardness are also very relevant in relating it to the severity of any head injury found.

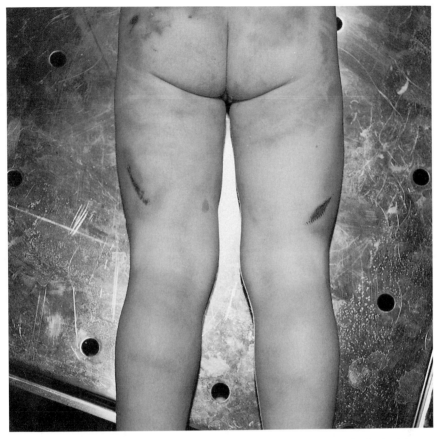

Figure 9.2 Abrasions found on a child, who was the victim of multiple fatal non-accidental injuries. These matched the edge of a wooden toilet seat. The marks were caused by the child being forcibly pushed onto the seat.

supplied hot water to the sink and the bath, was made by a gas official. He concluded that, although the heater was working properly, the temperature of the water leaving the hot tap was too hot without mixing it with cold water. He also commented that the method of mixing was crude and should not be relied on for bathing.

In addition to the examination of specific items and surfaces, it is essential for the investigator to take note of the child's environment as a whole, i.e., the general appearance of the home, state of repair, degree of cleanliness, quality of clothing, food present and state of basic amenities.

The boundaries of a scene or scenes in child abuse, because of the multiplicity and varying ages of injury in many cases, may be difficult or impossible to define. One should be guided by accounts available relating to circumstances surrounding the episode leading to death together with the post-mortem findings.

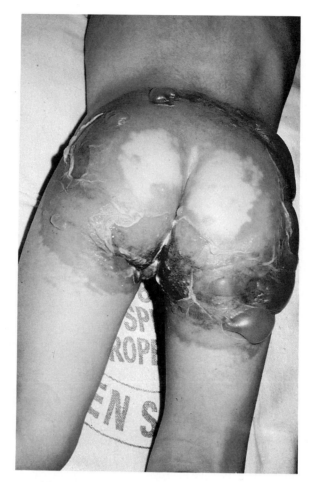

Figure 9.3(a) Scald marks on a child's buttock area showing tide marks and central spared areas caused by being held down in a bath containing hot water.

The scene and sudden death in infancy syndrome (SIDS)

Though there has been a major decrease over the last two years in the incidence of SIDS cases, in most Western countries it is still the most common cause of infant mortality in the first 12 months of life. In this age group, unnatural deaths, including homicides, are infrequent and may be missed initially. It is essential, therefore, in all cases where the manner of death is not obvious to cultivate a high index of suspicion tempered with a sensitive approach to the bereaved family. In all cases, however, where there is the slightest suspicion, the scene needs to be carefully evaluated (Iyasu et al., 1994).

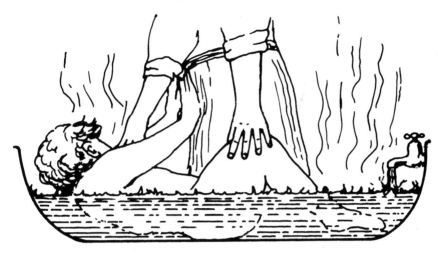

Figure 9.3(b) Diagram of the probable position in which the child was held in the bath. The hot water tap was turned on after the child was placed in the bath and held forcibly.

Bass et al. (1986) showed the need for caution in sudden infant death cases. They conducted death scene investigations in 26 consecutive cases in which a presumptive diagnosis of SIDS was made. In six cases they found strong circumstantial evidence of accidental death. In 18 other cases they discovered various possible causes of death other than SIDS, including accidental asphyxiation by an object in the cot, smothering by overlaying while sharing a bed, hyperthermia and shaken baby syndrome. Their study suggested that many sudden deaths of infants have a definable cause that can be revealed by careful investigation of the scene of death.

In any investigation of a SIDS death the following matters should always be specifically addressed:

1. Findings at the actual time that the baby was discovered dead.
2. Physical and socio-economic findings in the household within which the child has been living.
3. Immediate past medical history of the child.
4. Information about the parents and other siblings.
5. Full history of the child's developmental progress since birth.
6. Information about other current and previous members of the same household, including baby sitters and child minders.

At the scene one should take into account the following:

1. When and in what position, where and by whom was the child found dead?
2. Was there any vomit at the nostrils or mouth?
3. One should always examine the crib, cot or bed in which the child has been found dead, and take careful notes of any wetness thereon due to secretions, vomitus, etc. Any soiled bedding or baby clothes may have to be retained if this is felt appropriate. There is still some uncertainty as to whether the mattress may be of importance in relation to the causation of the death (i.e., the presence of fungal growth on it), and this may have to be kept (Blair et al., 1995). If it is felt that there

is a possibility that the design of the cot may have accounted for an accidental asphyxial death, this should also be retained and examined fully within the laboratory.

4.   One should take into account the general state of cleanliness of the house and other factors, which indicate lifestyle, socio-economic factors and provision for adequate nourishment for the family.

5.   Together with (4), one should also take into account the finding of any noxious substances, medicines, drugs of abuse, etc.

Accidental deaths in children with particular reference to asphyxia

There are many potential areas of danger in the home, particularly for the small child. It is essential to ascertain, when a child dies in a domestic environment as discussed above, the type of environment and conditions in which it is found. Accidents in the home may need careful differentiation from homicidal modes of death. If, for example, the child has died from poisoning, the availability of drugs and other

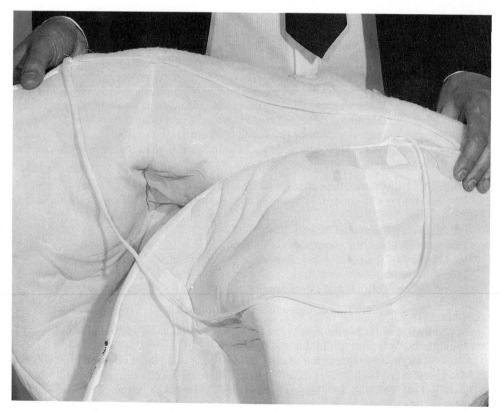

Figure 9.4(a)   The lining of a duvet showing the section that had become detached.

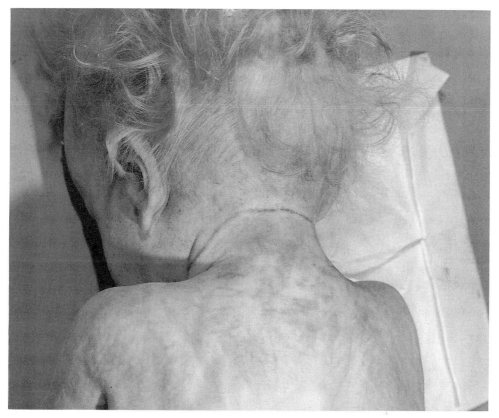

Figure 9.4(b) A view of a ligature mark around the child's neck, caused by the lining of the duvet becoming wound round the neck and causing constriction as the child struggled in vain to free itself.

harmful substances should be ascertained. Could a small child, for example, find carelessly placed medicines and take them of its own accord or was it deliberately poisoned?

Deaths involving mechanical asphyxia in particular, need to be carefully differentiated from those which are homicidal. The true manner of causation may be difficult to explain without thorough examination of the scene. Shepherd (1990) described an accidental self-strangulation in a 3-year-old child. The neck was compressed by a flex from a lamp, which had a heavy glass base and was situated on the window sill approximately level with the top of the bed. The author was able to reconstruct events by scene examination, which strongly suggested that the child's right arm had become entangled with the flex, and looped around the neck as the child turned over. Hanging in young children, as reported by Cooke et al. (1989), may occur in relation to the child's sleeping environment from mishaps involving the cot, its bedding or in conjuction with restraining straps. The latter authors found 11 deaths in children due to hanging. Similar cases were also reported by Variend and Usher (1984), who pointed out the inherent danger of putting infants in broken or modified cots, which do not conform to accepted standards.

CASE 9.3
A 12-month-old male infant was found dead with his neck entangled within a partially detached length of the lining of its duvet cover shown in Figure 9.4(a). A few blood stains mixed with saliva are also seen on the duvet. The child died as a result of accidental ligature strangulation (Figure 9.4(b)).

References

Bass M., Kravath R.E. and Class I. (1986) Death scene investigation in sudden infant death. *N. Engl. J. Med.* **315**, 100–105.

Blair P., Fleming P., Bensley D., Smith I., Bacon C. and Taylor E. (1995). Plastic matresses and sudden infant death syndrome (letter). *Lancet* **345**, 720.

Cameron J.M., Johnson H.R.M. and Camps F.E. (1966) The battered child syndrome. *Med. Sci. Law* **6**, 2–21.

Cooke C.T., Cadden G.A. and Hilton J.M.N. (1989) Hanging deaths in children. *Am. J. For. Med. Pathol.* **10**, 98–104.

Iyasu S., Hanslick R., Rowley D. and Wilinger M. (1994) Proceedings of Workshop on Guidelines for Scene Investigation of Sudden Unexplained Infant Deaths. *J. For. Sci.* **39**, 1126–1136.

Shepherd R.T. (1990) Accidental self-strangulation in a young child. *Med. Sci. Law* **30**, 119–123.

Variend S. and Usher A. (1984) Broken cots and infant fatality. *Med. Sci. Law* **24**, 111–112.

Wagner G.N. (1986) Crime scene investigation in child-abuse cases. *Am. J. For. Med. Pathol.* **7**, 94–99.

CHAPTER 10

Scene type: asphyxial and related deaths

Asphyxial and related deaths form an important group that can be categorised in a number of ways. For the purpose, however, of relating such deaths to scene examination, it is useful, from the practical point of view, to divide them into two broad groups, namely *mechanical* and *non-mechanical asphyxias*. The term mechanical, as used in this context, is a general term taken to mean that the flow of air into the body is physically compromised in some way, e.g., strangulation, traumatic asphyxia, choking; whereas non-mechanical relates to a physiological impediment to the uptake of oxygen by the body, e.g., carbon monoxide poisoning.

In addition, certain types of death which involve compression of the neck, although not predominantly asphyxial, are also included. These are cases where death does not result predominantly from deprivation of oxygen but rather from a cardio-inhibitory mechanism resulting from vagal stimulation.

It is not the intention of the authors to give a comprehensive account of asphyxial deaths but rather to highlight the various types seen where scene examination is particularly of value. Indeed, in some cases, the true nature of certain types of asphyxial deaths may be difficult to elucidate without a thorough scene examination.

Mechanical asphyxia and related deaths

AUTO-EROTIC DEATHS, PRINCIPALLY FROM ASPHYXIA

The scene in such deaths should be examined with care in order to establish:

1. Whether the death was due to the deceased's own actions or whether a third party was involved.
2. If a third party was involved, whether there was any intention to harm the victim.
3. Whether the asphyxia was, in fact, auto-erotic or whether there was some other explanation.

Figures 10.1 and 10.2 show two typical auto-erotic hanging deaths.

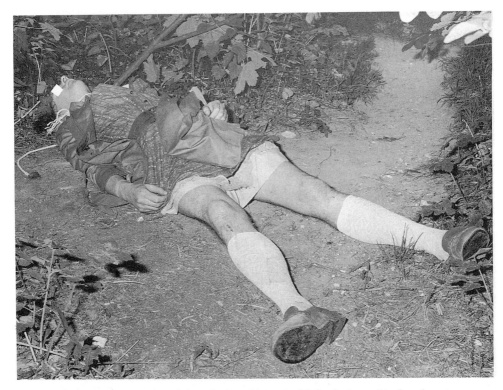

Figure 10.1 A young adult male found lying on his back dressed in female attire. He has a rope around his neck, which had been looped over the branch of an adjacent tree. The rope snapped after he had accidentally hanged himself. Note the ties around both wrists, which were connected to the other end of the rope in order to control the degree of neck compression.

Resnick (1972) was one of the first to enumerate the features, which are typical of this category of asphyxial death, which he called 'eroticized repetitive hanging syndrome'. These are:

1. They involve adolescent or young men (not exclusively and occasionally such deaths are also seen in females).
2. Ropes, belts or other binding material are found, and so arranged that compression of the neck may be produced and controlled voluntarily.
3. Evidence of masturbation.
4. Partial or complete nudity.
5. A solitary act.
6. Repetitive behaviour with attempts by the deceased to ensure that no visible marks are left on his person.
7. No apparent wish to die.
8. Binding of the body and/or extremities and/or genitals with ropes, chains or leather (less frequently).
9. Female attire may be present.

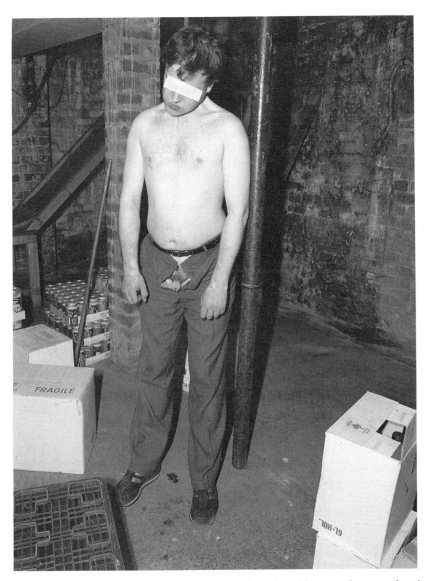

Figure 10.2 A young adult male, partially clothed, found hanging from overhead piping in a liquor store cellar where he worked. His trousers are open exposing his penis. In this case the deceased was able to control the degree of asphyxia with his feet touching the floor and bending slightly to allow further pressure to act on his neck structures. Nearby, is seen a red plastic crate, which he had used to reach the overhead pipe in order to tie and untie the rope.

One should also add to Resnick's list, the frequent finding of sexual aids such as pornographic material.

Garza-Leal and Landron (1991) describe a case where auto-erotic asphyxia was initially misinterpreted as suicidal and required careful reconstruction to arrive at the true manner of death. The deceased, who was partially suspended by a loop bound to his neck and left wrist, was cut down by his father in order to assist him. At that stage the scene investigators considered it a classic case of suicide and sent the body to the mortuary for autopsy. After the autopsy was carried out, the pathologists concluded that the manner of death did not fit in with a suicide. A scene reconstruction was then carried out using a doll and with information supplied by the father. The latter related that the body had been partially suspended by a noose around the neck, which passed around the horizontal rod of a closet, and that the other end of the noose was tied to the left wrist. The horizontal rod showed multiple previous abrasions. The body, according to the father, had also been gagged and was partially naked, with the legs crossed and tied by a bandage with a velcro clasp. He also admitted removing some pornographic pictures, which were on the floor in front of the body.

Scene reconstruction was also particularly relevant in a case involving siblings who died 18 years apart (Bell et al., 1991). They found that both the brothers, aged 13 and 24 years at the time of their deaths, were found partially naked and wearing female undergarments. Whereas one brother used only a belt, the other used an elaborate ligature consisting of a telephone cord and camera strap that enabled him to control the degree of neck compression.

In two cases described by O'Halloran and Dietz (1993), the victims had used hydraulic shovels on their tractors to suspend themselves. One of the deceased had even grown very fond of his vehicle, giving it a name and composing poetry for it.

Byard and Bramwell (1988) and Byard et al. (1990, 1993) made an analysis of the death scene features in a number of cases of female sexual asphyxias, and point out that, in females, the scene is less demonstrative of a sexual motive.

Although the most common type of auto-erotic asphyxia involves the use of a ligature to compress the neck, occasionally variants are seen as in the following case involving partial smothering. This type is much more unusual, and can initially be problematical in assessing whether or not foul play is involved.

CASE 10.1
In this case the deceased, a 54-year-old married man, had died from self-smothering caused by obstructing his nose and mouth. He frequently travelled away from home on business and was found dead in a hotel bedroom, wrapped in insulating tape, which covered both his trunk and most of his head (Figure 10.3). Beneath the tape on his head he wore a plastic bag with holes cut out for his mouth and eyes. In addition, he covered his head with one of the bed covers and secured it with tape. The wrapping around of the trunk was achieved, by firstly placing two black bin liners over his trunk so that they covered his chest and arms. He then secured one end of the tape to the nearby radiator pipe and then wrapped himself around the tape till it was used up. He was able with his hands, which were free, to place the central core of the tape reel over his penis. Clearly the elaborate nature of 'wrapping up' indicated that either someone had helped him or he had carried this out entirely by himself, having, through previous similar practice, 'perfected' the technique to the extent seen at death. Reconstruction of events by a volunteer (with appropriate safety precautions) showed that he could have achieved the 'wrapping up' entirely by himself. At the inquest the deceased's wife elaborated on her husband's proclivities in this direction and his unsuccesful attempts to encourage her participation.

Other types of auto-erotic deaths involve, for example, the use of objects for penetration, usually via the anus, such as a vacuum cleaner (Imami and Kemal,

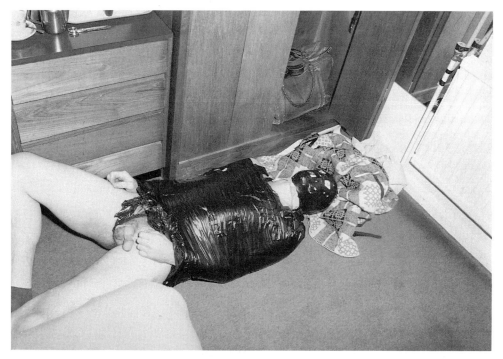

Figure 10.3 A middle-aged man shown lying in his hotel room wrapped with black insulating tape. Radiator piping shows part of tape attached. Bedding, which had covered the head, has been lifted off his face.

1988); electricity to heighten sexual arousal (Sivaloganathan, 1981; Tan and Chao, 1983); solvent sniffing (Bass, 1970); amyl nitrite (Louria, 1970; Sarvesvaran et al., 1992); partial drowning (Sivaloganathan, 1984). Examination of the deceased *in situ* in cases where death is not just a straightforward auto-erotic asphyxia involving a neck ligature, is essential. Indeed, the pathologist may not be able to arrive at the correct cause and mode of death without consideration of the scene environment in the first instance.

SUICIDAL HANGING

Most people hang themselves at home (Bowen, 1982; Davison and Marshall, 1986). Other frequently encountered locations include custodial environments, such as police cells and prisons, places of work, hospitals and secluded outdoor environments. In the latter situation the person may not be found for a considerable length of time after death.

There may be concern when the deceased is not found in the 'usual' hanging position. Many people are not aware that death from hanging may occur with virtually all of the deceased's body touching the floor. Indeed, occasionally such cases are misinterpreted as auto-erotic even though there is no other supportive evidence. Luke et al. (1985) and Davison and Marshall (1986) found that, in the majority of cases (53.3 and 59 per cent, respectively), some part of the body was touching the ground. Luke et al. further observed that in 43 per cent the feet were touching the ground and, in a smaller, but significant proportion, the body was supported either at knee or buttock level.

Examination of the scene will enable the investigator to appreciate the ease with which death from hanging may occur from easily accessible and low points of attachment. One must also look for any objects or items of furniture that would facilitate hanging, such as a chair, which may be pushed away to effect suspension. The point of attachment of the rope should be examined as well as the surrounding area. There may be disturbance of dust caused by the ligature being attached, particularly if it is a high point such as a beam. Corresponding dirt marks may be found on the hands or clothing of the deceased.

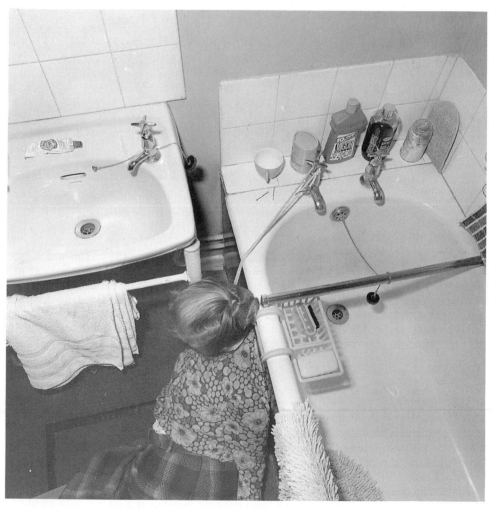

Figure 10.4 An elderly woman shown in the position in which she was found, with the lower part of her body touching the bathroom floor. The flex is seen extending from the right side of her neck to the bath tap.

CASE 10.2
A 76-year-old female suffering from terminal cancer was found lying on her bathroom floor (Figure 10.4). She had attached one end of an insulated electric flex to a bath tap and the other end was wound round her neck. She placed a piece of towelling between the ligature and her neck. It appears that the weight required to compress her neck was caused by the deceased allowing herself to fall forward against the pull of the flex.

SIMULATED SUICIDAL HANGING

A body may be suspended in order to mimic a suicidal hanging in cases where the deceased has been killed by a third party. Scene examination in such cases may be problematical unless meticulous attention is paid to the post-mortem examination, particularly to the type and distribution of injuries to the neck region. The scene may at first give no cause for concern and, indeed, as in the following case, there may be signs which are suggestive of suicide.

CASE 10.3
A 32-year-old female was found hanging from a bannister as shown in Figure 10.5(a) and (b). The relevant signs near the body, which could be interpreted as supporting a suicidal hanging, were a photograph of a middle-aged lady who presumably could have been a close relative, possibly her mother, and a telephone with its receiver off the hook. Did she try to phone a close friend or relative before hanging herself, with the photograph of a loved one nearby? The true explanation is quite different. She received a kick to the neck by her husband (Figure 10.5(c)), was then dragged to where she was found (the clothing has ridden up as a result of being dragged by the arms) and partially suspended by the bannister. The position of the telephone receiver resulted from her daughter discovering her mother, trying to phone for help, then dropping the receiver and running around to a next-door neighbour. Furthermore, the photograph, when examined closely, was, in fact, an advertisement for hair styling.

In *R. v. Emmett-Dunne*, (General Court Martial at Dusseldorf, Germany) (Camps 1959), the killer murdered his victim by delivering a blow to the neck with the side of the hand, then suspended the body with the help of an accomplice. The pathological evidence found in the neck structures, namely a vertical fracture to the body of the thyroid cartilage as well as vertical tears to both carotid arteries, was incompatible with death occurring by hanging and thus incompatible with the position in which the deceased was found at the scene.

HOMICIDAL HANGING

Puschel et al. (1984) describe six cases of homicidal hanging and point out that distinguishing between murder and suicide may be impossible by examination of the body alone. It is essential to carry out a detailed investigation of the scene, reconstruction of the position of the suspended body, examination of the rope, the knots and the direction of the fibres on the rope. The body may have been incapacitated in some way, e.g., through drink or drugs, in order to effect hanging. Furthermore, it may be relatively easy to achieve if the assailant is a fit healthy person and the victim, very young, infirmed and/or elderly. Nevertheless, it has to be stated that this mode of homicide is rare.

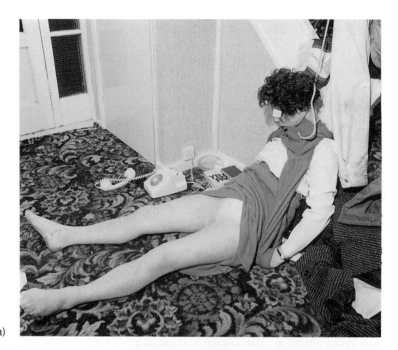

(a)

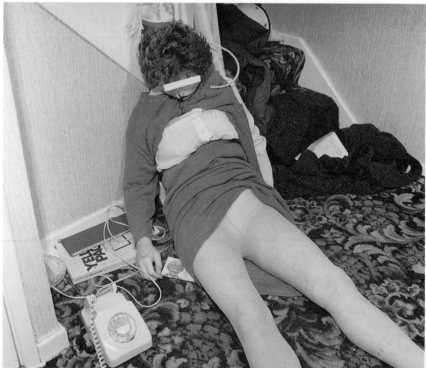

(b)

Figure 10.5(a) and **(b)** Two views of a woman who had been kicked in the neck by her husband and then suspended with a rope to a bannister to simulate suicide.

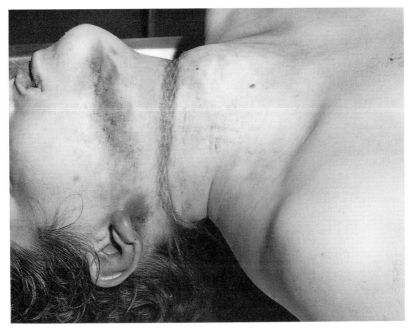

(c)

Figure 10.5(c) Once the neck had been extended, widespread bruising could be seen on the right side of the neck above the ligature mark.

SUICIDAL LIGATURE STRANGULATION

In the case described by Frazer and Rosenberg (1983), initially the authors considered the possibility that death was due to an auto-erotic asphyxia. The deceased, a 53-year-old white male, was found on the basement floor of his home in a kneeling position, wearing pyjamas, with the pyjama pants positioned at his hips. He had a ball of twine nearby with succesive layers of it wrapped around his neck, with the free end wrapped around his right thumb. Careful examination of the scene, however, showing an absence of pornographic material and other paraphenalia, as well as the absence of an 'escape mechanism', supported their contention that the death was suicidal. The deceased had, in fact, wrapped the twine around his neck 35 times; multiple encircling of the neck being a common feature of suicidal ligature strangulation.

SMOTHERING

With homicidal smothering, careful examination of a scene is essential, especially where death may involve the elderly, infirmed or very young and there are very few signs of disturbance. Any items which may have been used for smothering, such as a pillow or bedding, need to be collected and examined for saliva, blood, hair and other trace evidence, which could have been transferred from the deceased (Figure 10.6). A pillow, for example, may also show an obvious indentation where it has been pressed over the face. This must be photographed before removal. In very young children the bedding in the cot needs to be carefully examined.

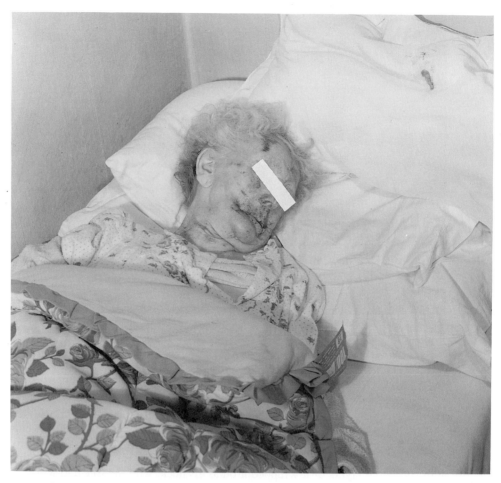

Figure 10.6 An elderly woman lying face up in bed. Note the scratch marks and bruises to the face and the indentation, blood and other fluid stains on the pillow, which had been forced over her face to smother her.

In the following case, the deceased was smothered as a result of his face being pushed into soft earth.

CASE 10.4
A 55-year-old male was found dead, lying face down in woodland. The ground on which he was found was noted to be very soft underfoot. When the body was turned over a pronounced indentation of the soil was seen where his face had been. On examination in the mortuary it was established that there was a substantial amount of mud present in the mouth and eyes. In addition the forehead, near the midline was abraided. Furthermore, on dissecting the back of the neck, bruising was found within the musculature of the back of the head and upper neck, indicating that he had been pushed down hard into the soft earth from behind (Figure 10.7(a)–(d)).

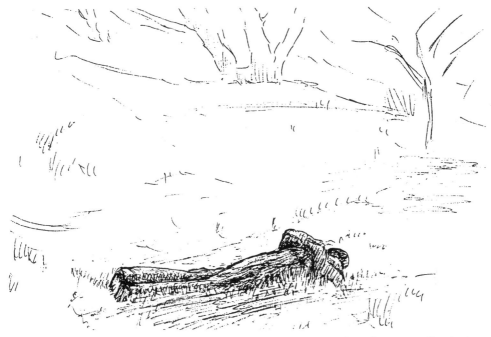

Figure 10.7(a) An adult male shown lying face down in soft earth in a woodland.

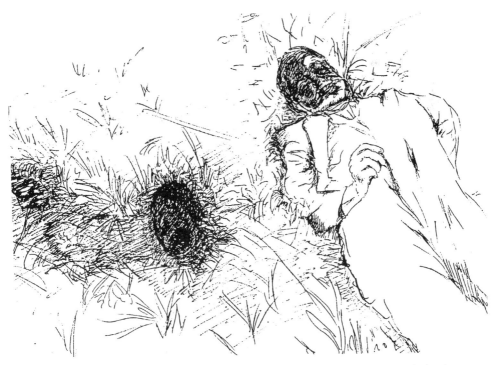

Figure 10.7(b) Once the body had been turned over, the indentation made by the deceased's face, which had been pushed hard into the ground, is evident. In addition, one can see that the central area has a deeper indentation caused by his nose.

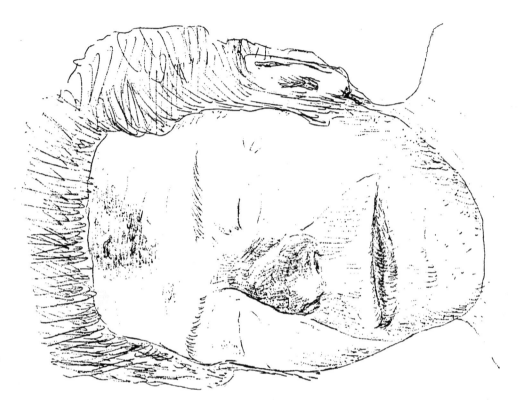

Figure 10.7(c)   Once the face had been cleaned, grazing can be seen on the forehead and nose, caused by forcing the face down into the ground.

Suicidal smothering by means of a pillow is very unusual but has been described by Hicks et al. (1990) in a chronically mentally ill patient. The death scene in this case was a major part of the investigation, which enabled homicide to be ruled out.

SUFFOCATION WITH A PLASTIC BAG

A plastic bag may have been used for suffocation and, unless it is still in position over the face, it will be extremely difficult to reach the conclusion that death has resulted from this method. If the bag had been recently removed prior to discovery, there may be an inappropriate degree of condensation found on the face. In addition, in cases where the bag had been covering the face for some time, the degree of putrefactive change to the face may be accelerated in relation to other exposed parts of the body. Occasionally, if the bag had been placed tightly around the neck, a ligature mark may be found. The use of a plastic bag together with drugs has been a method favoured for assisted suicide cases. A careful search of the scene in such cases may reveal tablets and/or containers as well as literature on assisted suicide.

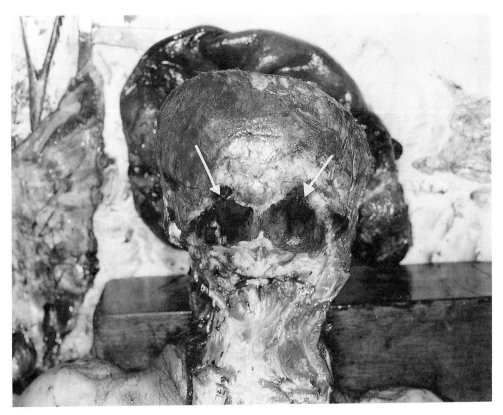

Figure 10.7(d)   The skin and subcutaneous tissue of the back of the neck has been reflected and dissected off to reveal the underlying musculature between the base of the skull and the upper neck. Within the muscle, bruising can be seen, which has been caused by pushing the back of the deceased's head and neck hard into the ground.

CASE 10.5
An elderly couple were found lying dead on top of their bed fully dressed. The scene was not disturbed in any way and indeed the room was clean and tidy. A variety of different tablets and containers were found in the kitchen, some of which were empty. The woman had died from a drugs overdose cocktail whereas her husband had died by placing a plastic bag over his face, which he secured with a ligature (no traces of any drugs were found in him). It appears that the couple had clearly planned to end their lives. However, it was not possible to assess whether the woman had taken the overdose before her husband killed himself and, furthermore, there were no indications that the couple had been assisted by a third party to end their lives (Figures 10.8(a)–(c)).

POSTURAL ASPHYXIA

In such cases, it is essential to appreciate that asphyxia has resulted from the position of the body causing some form of restriction of the airway. Almost invariably there are predisposing factors, such as alcohol, drug abuse or some form of infirmity.

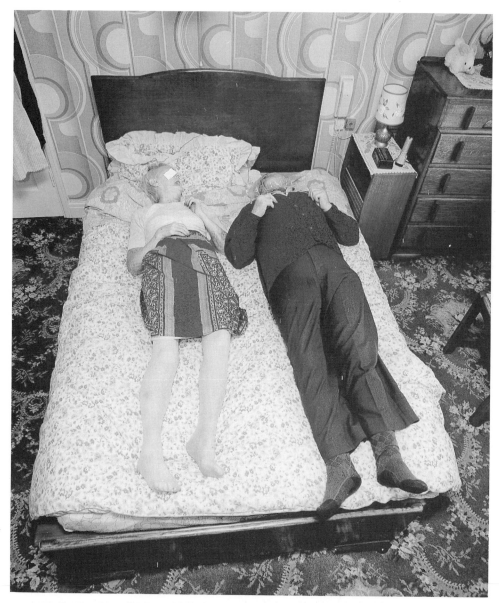

Figure 10.8(a) A view of an elderly couple as they were found lying on their bed.

Careful assessment of the scene in relation to body position is essential in order to allow correct interpretation of the autopsy findings. In a recent study (Bell et al., 1991), 30 cases were assessed. They found chronic alcoholism or acute alcohol intoxication to be a significant factor in 75 per cent with an average blood alcohol of 240 mg/100 ml. Victims were commonly found in a restrictive position producing hyperflexion of the head and neck.

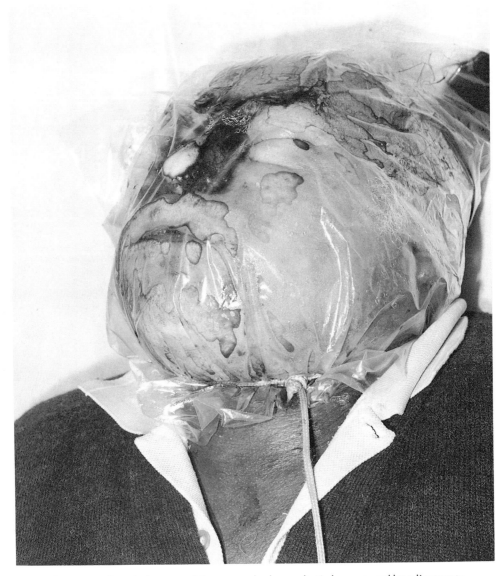

Figure 10.8(b)   A close-up of the man, who has a plastic bag secured by a ligature to the neck. Note that the body shows signs of decomposition.

It is important to differentiate such cases from those due to other causes in which the deceased is found face down with florid hypostasis in the dependent areas accompanied by coarse petechial haemorrhages within these areas. The petechial haemorrhages in such circumstances are produced after death. The most difficult cases to assess are those where the head is found at a lower level than the trunk and there is gross congestion to the upper part of the chest, head and neck. The following is such an example.

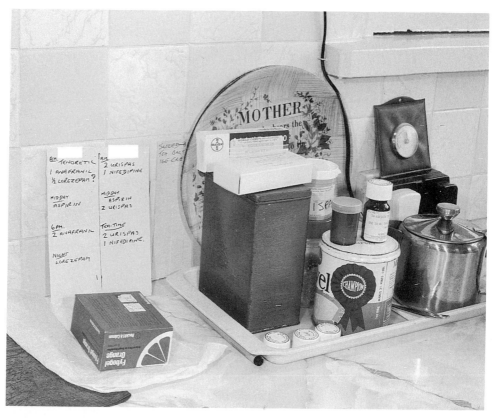

Figure 10.8(c)   Some of the many tablets found in the couple's flat.

CASE 10.6

The deceased, a 26-year-old female, was found dead slumped over the side of the bed as shown in Figure 10.9(a). Detailed examination of the body *in situ* revealed that her head, neck and part of her upper chest were hanging over the side. The hypostasis and intense congestion of the head in particular, were typical of this part of the body being lowermost. The deceased also had extensive petechial haemorrhages of the face and eyes. All haemorrhages were within the area of hypostasis. The face was also somewhat swollen due to intense congestion with blood (Figure 10.9(b)). There had undoubtedly been some pressure from the side of the bed onto the front of the neck because of the blanched area at the front of the neck (Figure 10.9(c)). Internal examination of the body revealed areas of confluent petechial haemorrhages in the scalp, which may be easily confused with bruising occasioned by impacts; the bleeding, however, was symmetrical. Bruising to the muscles of the front of the neck was exaggerated and much of it probably artefactual. There was no fracture to the larynx or hyoid bone. She was found to have significant drugs (dipipanone and diazepam) in her body to have caused her to have at least become unconscious. Just prior to her death she had been involved in sexual activity, although the nature of this was not clear. The dilemma here is an obvious one. Did the deceased succumb to compression of her neck from a third party or could all the findings be explained on the basis of the position in which she was found

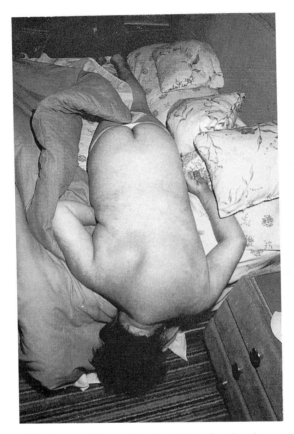

Figure 10.9(a)   The deceased shown *in situ* with her head and upper trunk hanging down from the side of the bed.

at the scene together with incapacitation from drugs? Since all the findings can be explained on the latter basis and, bearing in mind that, on the surface of her neck, no external injuries associated with compression were found, then the latter mode of death appears highly likely.

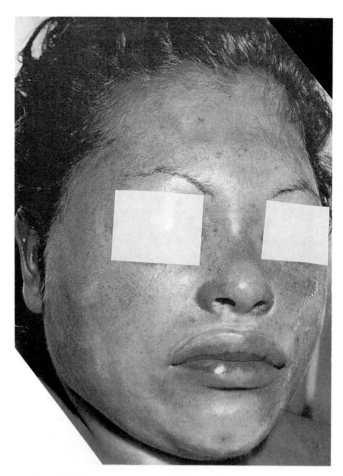

Figure 10.9(b) The face is swollen and intensely congested. Numerous petechial haemorrhages can also be seen.

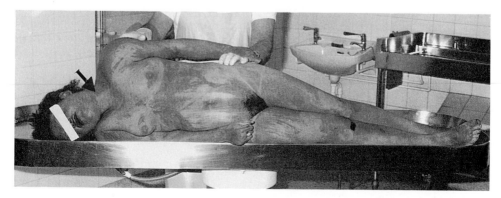

Figure 10.9(c) The front of the body showing distribution of the hypostasis. The front of the neck is blanched where it had been pressed against the side of the bed.

Deaths resulting from a vitiated atmosphere, or the presence of irrespirable or toxic gases

CARBON MONOXIDE POISONING

When investigating the cause of a carbon monoxide poisoning, potential sources of the gas must be identified and tested individually to find out which of them is responsible for its production. This testing must be carried out at the scene of the incident in order that the conditions under which the poisoning took place can be replicated (Health and Safety Executive, 1984); it is often a combination of circumstances rather than a specific fault that causes a fatality. Inevitably there will be aspects of the scene that cannot be reproduced, most frequently the weather conditions. However, efforts must be made to find out from those who first entered the premises: whether doors and windows were open or closed; the status of the appliances that are to be tested; the location and last reported movements of the victims; and the length of time over which exposure to fumes could have taken place. Enquiries may also reveal a history or pattern of occurrence of symptoms, which clearly reflects intermittent exposure over a period of time. The first onset sometimes coincides with a change to the structure or contents of the premises being examined, with individual episodes arising from specific activities or conditions.

At the scene of a carbon monoxide poisoning, bodies should be examined and removed before any tests are carried out. The victim's location should be noted so that gas samples can be taken from that area during the test and, as CO poisoning can induce nausea, the presence of any vomit in the premises should also be noted, it may indicate that the victim moved before final collapse. The body itself should be visually examined. Carboxyhaemoglobin introduces a distinctive bright-red coloration to the blood and this may be apparent if hypostasis is visible. It is advisable that on-site CO measurements should only be carried out after it has been confirmed by toxicological analysis that carbon monoxide poisoning was indeed the cause of death. Each suspect appliance in the premises should be carefully inspected. Inefficient combustion produces particulate carbon as well as CO and the presence of heavy soot deposits in heater assemblies, warm air vents and flues will indicate the appliance that is likely to be the source of the problem.

Exhaust fumes from internal combustion engines contain very high concentrations of CO, which can rapidly cause death if inhaled within an enclosed space. The deliberate introduction of fumes into the interior of a car by means of a pipe attached to the exhaust or by running the engine in a closed garage is a common method of suicide. Accidental death can also occur in the latter circumstances if the victim is unaware of the toxic nature of exhaust gases or fails to make adequate provision for ventilation when working on a vehicle. The cause of such deaths may be readily apparent from an inspection of the car and its surroundings – the ignition will be switched on and the victim lying in an enclosure where exhaust fumes can accumulate – but there may be occasions where there appears to be adequate ventilation at the scene, or a very brief exposure and CO levels have to be measured. If a car engine is allowed to idle in an enclosed space, carbon deposits will accumulate in the cylinders and on the spark plugs as the air is exhausted and the engine will eventually stall. As it is unlikely that the victim would turn off the ignition before succumbing to the fumes, any electrical equipment remaining switched on may have left the battery flat.

Before any tests are carried out the battery should be recharged, the plugs cleaned and the car driven for a few miles to burn off the carbon deposits. The car can then be tested in a condition that more nearly replicates its state at the time of the incident. There have been reports of fires occurring in cars used for suicide attempts where a hose has been attached to the exhaust. The precise mechanism by which such fires start is currently unclear.

ASHYXIA FROM OTHER GASES

Byard and Wilson (1992) describe two cases of methane asphyxia occurring in boys of 11 and 12 years who were found at the bottom of a 37 ft (11.1 m) deep sewer shaft. Analysis of the gas in the shaft revealed 21 per cent oxygen at the surface, 14.3 per cent at a depth of 5 ft (1.5 m) and only 4.8 per cent at depths of 10 ft (3 m) and below. Other gases detected at lower levels were methane, nitrogen and carbon dioxide (4.3 per cent). These cases demonstrate the value of atmospheric gas analysis in cases of possible methane asphyxia in confirming the presence of methane and in demonstrating levels of oxygen below that necessary to support life.

Manning et al. (1981) discuss the importance of proper scene investigation in order to enable one to arrive at the correct cause of death. They describe the deaths of three men who descended into an open drainage pit to recover a fallen grate lid. Each man in turn was immediately overcome and died within minutes of his descent. Initial analysis of the pit's air indicated a methane level of 15 per cent. It was therefore initially assumed that death was due to methane poisoning. Post-mortem analysis of the victim's tissues, however, yielded methane levels in only faint trace quantities (0–100 µg/100 g range). Analysis of the air samples taken at various pit levels revealed that, as one descended, there was a decrease in oxygen levels, from 20 per cent at the top to 3 per cent at the bottom. CO_2 levels, however, increased from the top of the pit, and reached a level of 22 per cent at the 6 ft depth of the pit. The accepted lethal level is only 10 per cent. The cause originally attributed to these deaths was shown to be in error.

Downs et al. (1994), describe two suicides, one resulting from carbon dioxide in the form of dry ice and the other from the use of propane gas. They emphasise the importance of environmental sampling. One should add that, as with all cases where the atmosphere is potentially hazardous, appropriate protective clothing including full breathing apparatus will need to be worn.

References

Bass M. (1970) Sudden sniffing death. *JAMA* **212**, 2075–2079.
Bell M.D., Tate L.G. and Wright R.K. (1991) Sexual asphyxia in siblings. *Am. J. For. Med. Pathol.* **12**, 77–79.
Bowen D.A.L. (1982) Hanging – a review. *For. Sci. Int.* **20**, 247–249.
Byard R.W. and Bramwell N.H. (1988) Autoerotic death in females. An underdiagnosed syndrome? *Am. J. For. Med. Pathol.* **9**, 252–254.
Byard R.W. and Wilson G.W. (1992) Death scene gas analysis in suspected methane asphyxia. *Am. J. For. Med. Pathol.* **13**, 69–71.
Byard R.W., Hucker S.J. and Hazelwood R.R. (1990) A comparison of typical death scene features in cases of fatal male and autoerotic asphyxia with a review of the literature. *For. Sci. Int.* **48**, 113–121.

Byard R.W., Hucker S.J. and Hazelwood R.W. (1993) Fatal and near-fatal autoerotic asphyxial episodes in women. *Am. J. For. Med. Pathol.* **14**, 70–73.

Camps F.E. (1959) The case of Emmett-Dunne. *Med. Leg. J.* **27**, 156–161.

Davison A. and Marshall T.K. (1986) Hanging in Northern Ireland – a survey. *Med. Sci. Law* **26**, 23–28.

Downs J.C., Conradi S.E. and Nichols C.A. (1994) Suicide by environmental hypoxia (forced depletion of oxygen). *Am. J. For. Med. Pathol.* **15**, 216–223.

Frazer M. and Rosenberg S. (1983) A case of suicidal ligature strangulation. *Am. J. For. Med. Pathol.* **4**, 351–354.

Garza-Leal J.A. and Landron F.J. (1991) Autoerotic asphyxial death initially misinterpreted as suicide and a review of the literature. *J. For. Sci.* **36**, 1753–1759.

Health and Safety Executive (1984) *Carbon Monoxide.* Environmental Series Guidance Note EH 43. HMSO, London.

Hicks L.J., Scanlon M.J., Bostwick T.C. and Batten P.J. (1990) Death by smothering and its investigation. *Am. J. For. Med. Pathol.* **11**, 291–293.

Imami R.H. and Kemal M. (1988) Vacuum cleaner use in autoerotic death. *Am. J. For. Med. Pathol.* **9**, 246–248.

Louria D.B. (1970) Sexual use of amyl nitrite. *Med. Aspects Hum. Sex* **4**, 89.

Luke J.L., Reay D.T., Eisele J.W. and Bonnell H.J. (1985) Correlation of circumstances with pathological findings in asphyxial deaths by hanging: a prospective study of 61 cases from Seattle, WA. *J. For. Sci.* **30**, 1140–1147.

Manning T.J., Ziminnki K., Hyman A., Figueroa G. and Lukash L. (1981) Methane deaths? Was it the cause? *Am. J. For. Med. Pathol.* **2**, 333–336.

O'Halloran R.L. and Dietz P.E. (1993) Autoerotic fatalities with power hydraulics. *J. For. Sci.* **38**, 359–364.

Puschel K., Holtz W., Hidebrand E., Naeve W. and Brinkmann B. (1984) Hanging, suicide or homicide? [in German]. *Arch Kriminol.* **174**, 141–153.

Resnick H. (1972) Eroticized repetitive hanging: a form of self-destructive behavior. *Am. J. Psychother.* **26**, 4–21.

Sarvesvaran E.R., Fysh R. and Bowen D.A.L. (1992) Amyl nitrite related deaths. *Med. Sci. Law* **32**, 267–269.

Sivaloganathan S. (1981) Curiosum eroticum: a case of fatal electrocution during autoerotic practice. *Med Sci Law* **21**, 47–50.

Sivaloganathan S. (1984) Aqua-eroticum – a case of auto-erotic drowning. *Med. Sci. Law* **24**, 300–302.

Tan C.T.T. and Chao T.C. (1983) A case of fatal electrocution during an unusual autoerotic practice. *Med. Sci. Law* **23**, 92–95.

CHAPTER 11

The scene in other types of suspicious death

Falls

FALLS FROM A HEIGHT (OVER 10–12 FEET)

Falls from high places usually come within the accidental or suicidal category; only very occasionally are they shown to occur as a result of a homicidal act. Furthermore, one should also bear in mind the possibility that a dead body may be cast off the edge of a building, for example, and sustain post-mortem injuries, which need to be carefully evaluated and differentiated from those that may have occurred before death. An extensive study of the type and distribution of injuries seen in falls was made by Goonetilleke (1980).

When someone is found dead with multiple injuries near a high-rise building or other place where a fall could have occurred, careful reconstruction of the scene in conjunction with the post-mortem findings is essential in order to ascertain whether:

- Fatal injuries were caused by a fall from a height.
- Fatal injuries were caused by some other means at ground level, e.g., severe beating or vehicular accident.
- The immediate environment of the body is where the injuries were sustained.
- There are other signs/injuries on the body, which indicate circumstances other than a fall.

Scene assessment

With respect to scene assessment, the following items need to be considered.

The place from where the person fell

The point from which the fall occurred, e.g., balcony or window, needs to be assessed carefully to ascertain its feasibility or likelihood of being the origin of the fall. The height of railings should be measured, and any marks on them documented and evaluated. The place from where the deceased is thought to have fallen should be assessed to ascertain whether it would have been accessible to the victim. Furthermore, it should be examined for any signs to indicate whether there had been a struggle with a third party, such as disturbance of furniture and other items, evidence of injury resulting in loss of blood, etc. There may also be evidence at the scene that the deceased had attempted another mode of suicide before jumping. There may be empty tablet containers, possibly an implement such as a knife with blood staining, which may account for the presence of incised wounds to the body caused prior to precipitation. The presence of a note indicating intent to commit suicide should always be looked for.

The scene of the fall should also be examined to assess whether the person could have fallen accidentally. There may be unsafe slippery surfaces, loose tiles or brickwork, or structures around the perimeter of a roof or balcony, for example, which have given way with the weight of a person's body.

The place where the body was found

Examination of the position of the body in relation to the distance from a high-rise buiding, the presence and distribution of blood stains, impact marks, etc. will help build up a picture of the type of fall and the distance through which the person fell. Rabl et al. (1990) describe the case of a 19-year-old man found in the middle of a road near a flyover. Initially homicide was suspected because there were some strange findings; his legs were crossed, and a cigarette stub was found between the fingers of the right hand and suspect head injuries. Further investigations revealed that the deceased had fallen from the flyover.

The route taken by the body to reach the ground

When a person falls, there may be contact against parts of the buiding on the way to the ground. Such secondary glancing impacts are very likely to leave marks on the body and/or clothing as well as deflect the body from its straightest downward course. It is important to examine the building in the line of fall, looking for damage to structures such as brickwork and contamination with body fluids, hair or other trace evidence from the deceased.

BALLOON ACCIDENTS

A discussion of falls from aircraft is beyond the scope of this text but it is worth noting briefly the following observations made in balloon accidents. Usually deaths in such cases result from blunt impact trauma from falling from a height and Aguilar (1980) described such an accident in which there were three fatalities. It should be appreciated that one of the most common ways in which such accidents occur is by powerline contact and McConnell et al. (1992) described a death, which resulted from electrocution rather than blunt trauma. Examination of the deceased showed electrical burns and the gondola revealed scuff marks on the leather rim resulting from contact with the powerline.

LOW FALLS (UNDER 10–12 FEET)

Such lower level falls, which may cause concern as to the manner of causation, principally form two groups: (1) falls from a higher level, descending to the point of final impact, for example, falling down a flight of stairs; and (2) falling from one's own height.

Falls down stairs

Someone found at the bottom of a flight of stairs may pose a number of questions for the investigator, the most obvious being whether or not the person was killed by the action of a third party.

Such an assessment can only be made by taking into account the following:

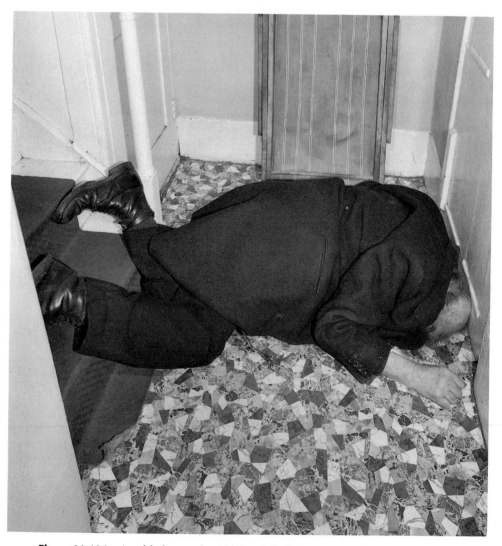

Figure 11.1(a) An elderly man found lying at the bottom of a flight of stairs with his head pressed against the cupboard door.

1. The presence of injuries to the body. If there are no injuries, then one should consider the possibility that the person died of natural causes and collapsed at the bottom of the stairs.
2. If there are injuries, whether they are consistent with falling or being propelled down stairs, bearing in mind the type of stairs, width, the number of flights involved, structure of stairs and walls, etc.
3. Possible evidence of a fight at, say, the top landing with the person receiving the most severe injuries there before falling.

All these possible scenarios should be going through the mind of the investigator and considered carefully during the course of the scene examination, and then, finally, assessed together with the pathologist's findings at the post-mortem examination.

CASE 11.1
An elderly man was found dead at home after the police were informed by a friend that he had not seen him for 3 days. The deceased was lying at the bottom of a flight of stairs as shown in Figure 11.1(a). The death was initially treated as suspicious because, when the detectives arrived at his house, no explanation was forthcoming as to why the door had been forced open (Figure 11.1(b)). It later transpired that this had been done by the first officer at the scene. After leaving the scene, he omitted to inform anyone that he had effected entry in this manner before going off duty for the weekend. The deceased it appears, had tripped and fallen forwards down the stairs, with his head impacting

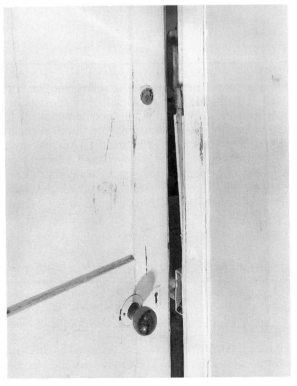

Figure 11.1(b) A view of the front door after forced entry.

against a cupboard door opposite the bottom stair. He died as a result of fracturing his cervical spine.

Epileptic deaths

In cases of sudden unexpected death from epilepsy there are frequently no specific anatomical findings seen at autopsy (Leestma et al., 1985). Occasionally, therefore, particularly if death has occurred in a young person and when it is not expected, it may be treated initially as suspicious. The deceased may, for example, die in bed with asphyxial changes because the face may have been pressed into a pillow. (Schwender and Troncoso (1986), in their series found that 23 out of 29 cases had been found dead in their bed or elsewhwere in the bedroom.) There may also be injuries from fits or the deceased may have fallen into a bath and drowned. Investigation of the scene can therefore be crucial in eliminating any suspicion of foul play in such circumstances as well as differentiating from other unnatural causes. The scene, particularly if there are injuries present, should be examined to assess where the deceased could have received such injuries in relation to the position of the body. Distribution of any blood and other body fluids and materials should also be noted; epileptics may bite their tongue, and lose blood and saliva from the mouth; lose bladder control and occasionally may also defecate. The house should also be searched for any medication.

Electrocution deaths

Wright (1983) states that proper investigation of injury and death from electrocution requires a high level of suspicion, as examination of the victim will often prove negative. There must be careful photographic documentation of the scene in every case. In low-voltage cases, the equipment that may have been involved should be photographed, X-rayed and examined electrically. Autopsy examination of the victim in cases of electrocution due to high-voltage alternating or direct current usually reveals burns and non-specific findings of asphyxia. Victims of low-voltage alternating current often have no electrical burns and the absence of findings, characteristic of ventricular fibrillation. Low-voltage direct current rarely produces death.

Fatalities involving stabbing or incised injuries

Stabbing is by far the most common method of homicide in the United Kingdom, and most cases are seen as a result of either domestic violence or the street or tavern brawl. It is uncommon to find the knife lying at the scene. In a domestic situation it may be cleaned up and put back in the kitchen drawer or disposed of. In street violence cases it is nearly always removed from the scene. The handling of the scene, blood distribution, etc. are dealt with elsewhere and case examples cited. Apart from dealing with the clearly homicidal cases, it is occasionally required to consider the question of whether the wound or wounds, be they stab or incised, were self-inflicted or indeed could have been accidental.

HOMICIDAL VERSUS SUICIDAL STABBING OR INCISED INJURIES

There are a number of considerations that the investigator must address when dealing with a stabbing, where the the possibility of suicide has been raised. Although it should be generally appreciated that, in some cases, this issue may never be resolved satisfactorily, there are a number of useful features of the scene, which, when considered together with other circumstances and the autopsy examination, lead one to the opinion that the injuries were self-inflicted.

Most suicidal stabbings occur in private. Start et al. (1992) in their series of 28 cases found only 2 (7 per cent) that were witnessed by other persons. Twenty-two (29 per cent) of the victims were found at their own home and, of these, the bedroom (nine cases) was the most common room, followed by the kitchen (six cases), bathroom and living room (three cases each) and garden (one case). It is of interest that eight (29 per cent) of the victims moved to a different room or location after the initial stabbing.

The weapon in nearly all cases is still at the scene and usually very close to the deceased or, occasionally, still in the hand or within a stab wound. One must also bear in mind that a well-meaning relative or friend may have removed the weapon.

The scene shows a lack of disturbance contrary to what one usually sees with homicidal cases and the door is frequently locked from the inside to ensure privacy.

Clothing should be carefully examined before the body is moved from the scene to see whether it has been altered in some way; suicidal stabbing victims frequently bare the area which is to be injured rather than stab through clothing.

Another excellent indicator of suicide is the presence of tentative marks. These are small multiple superficial cuts or puncture wounds to the body, usually grouped together in one or more areas and produced before the fatal injuries (Vanezis and West, 1983).

An unusual case is described by Schmidt et al. (1991) concerning a 47-year-old man, who was found dead at the bottom of a wall outside the door of the cellar of his house. He had a laceration to the scalp, an incised wound in front of the neck and several stab wounds to the left chest penetrating through clothing. Initially the death was highly suggestive of homicide. His wife related to the police that he was depressed, had inflicted the cutting injuries, made an unsuccesful attempt at self-strangulation and then finally jumped from a wall to the position where he was found. Post-mortem examination revealed wounds consistent with being self-inflicted, including hesitation marks to the left side of the neck.

The deceased may occasionally place himself in front of a mirror, as in the suicidal cut-throat case descibed below, and investigators should be aware of this possibility when assessing the manner of injury causation (Riddick et al., 1989).

CASE 11.2
The deceased, a 56-year-old man, was found in his bedroom lying on his bed as shown in Figure 11.2(a). There is a dressing-table mirror directly opposite where he had been sitting. A closer view of his clothing in Figure 11.2(b) shows that the blood had flowed downwards from the incised wounds to his neck. On the front of his trousers there is

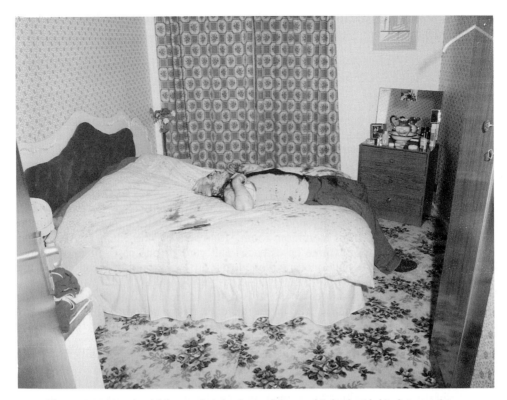

Figure 11.2(a)   A middle-aged male shown lying on his bed with his feet touching the floor and facing a dressing-table mirror.

relative absence of blood within areas previously creased as he had been sitting on the edge of the bed. A knife is present near his right hand. The room was tidy and the police had to force the lock to gain entry.

Deaths in the bath

When someone is found dead in a bath there are a number possibilities which one must be aware of:

1. Is the bath relevant to the death or is it coincidental?
2. Did the deceased get into the bath voluntarily and die thereafter, or did he/she fall in or was perhaps forced in?

Devos et al. (1985) in a retrospective study spanning 50 years found that 52 per cent were due to carbon monoxide poisoning, 20 per cent were suicides, 8.5 per cent were due to natural causes, 8.5 per cent were accidental drownings (mainly infants that were left unattended) and 6 per cent were homicides.

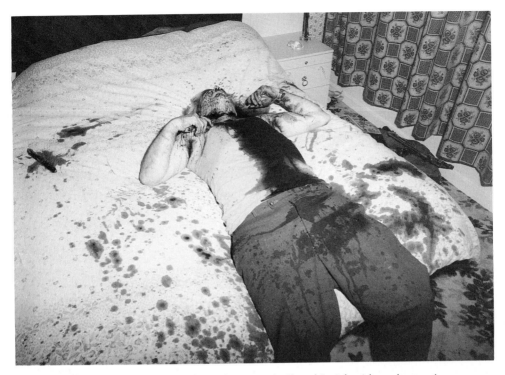

Figure 11.2(b)   A closer view showing a knife to his right side and extensive bloodstaining on both the deceased and the bed cover. The distribution of the bloodstaining clearly indicates that, when the injuries were inflicted, he was sitting on the edge of the bed before collapsing back.

EXAMINATION OF THE SCENE AND THE DECEASED IN SITU

Examination of the deceased *in situ*, the rest of the bathroom and, indeed, the other areas in the residence may provide valuable pointers to the forensic team as to the true nature of the death.

Initially, it is important to note whether there is water in the bath, and its depth and the degree to which the body is covered. The position of the head in relation to the water level may be relevant, particularly if one is considering drowning as a possibility (Figure 11.3). It should be appreciated, however, that, unless the body is discovered very early, the water level will fall and, indeed, may be very low or non-existent. This will be accelerated if water is leaking through the plug. It is helpful in such cases to establish where the original water level may have been by looking carefully for a possible line of deposit around the bath. This is particularly easy to see if the water is dirty. It is also important to measure the temperature of the water. The position of the plug itself should be noted. Did someone let the water out after death? It may also be relevant to retain a sample of water for analysis.

As far as the body is concerned, its position, whether prone or supine, should be noted as well as the position and angulation of the limbs. The presence, type and extent

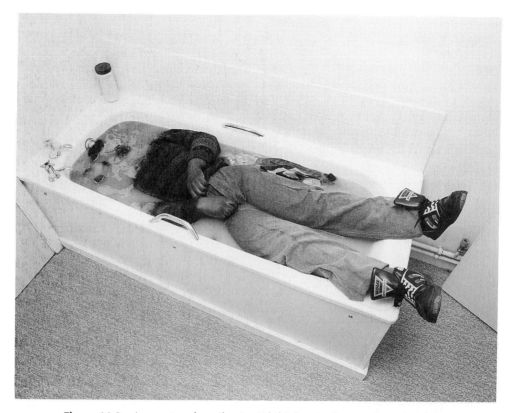

Figure 11.3 A young male epileptic with his head submerged in a half-filled bath tub.

of clothing, or any other coverings on the deceased should also be noted. It is also important to note the position of the taps and other objects attached to the bath and their relevance to any injuries on the body.

Examination of the bathroom should take into account how the water supply and room are heated. Whether there was a gas-fuelled heater and a possible source of carbon monoxide. Examination of the type of ventilation and its adequacy is important. The floor of the bath may be wet, particularly if there has been a struggle with spillage of water onto the floor. This may not be immediately obvious, particularly if the floor is carpeted and some time has passed. One would need to lift any top floor covering and note the dampness underneath.

CASE 11.3

A 64-year-old female was found lying on her right side in her bath. She was initially stabbed once in the back, knocked unconscious and then put into a bath half-filled with water, where she drowned. The bath water was contaminated with blood from the stabbing injury. On lifting the linoleum floor, which had been cleaned by the assailants, water was found underneath (Figure 11.4). The water had spilled onto the floor when they placed the deceased in the bath.

Hayman (1986) describe the case of a 42-year-old woman found in a bath, which

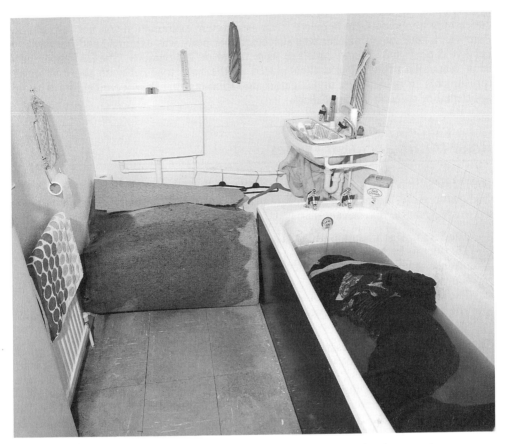

Figure 11.4   The deceased is shown *in situ* in the bath tub. The water is bloodstained, and the carpet has been lifted back to show that the linoleum floor and carpet had been soaked with water from splashing during the course of the assailant depositing the body into a half-filled bath.

was initially thought to be homicidal because the deceased had suffered a severe head injury. She was found fully clothed and submerged in water with her head lying over the bath plug. Both taps were turned on and water had overflowed into several adjacent rooms. Blood was spattered extensively over the bathroom tiles and adjacent sink, and on the inside of the plastic shower curtain. The deceased held a hammer loosely in her left hand, and underneath the bath plug was a prescription for a proprietary preparation containing carbromal and pentobarbitone. At post-mortem she was found to have two irregular lacerations, one in the centre of the forehead and the other at the occiput. No fractured skull was noted. She was found to have taken a barbiturate overdosage and the cause of death was given as drowning and pentobarbitone overdose. It appears that she had stood in the bath after taking a lethal overdose of the drug and battered herself repeatedly over the head with a hammer before losing consciousness and drowning.

Lasczkowski et al. (1992) report the case of a 65-year-old lady found dead in her bath and discuss the problems arising from the examination of bodies in such circumstances.

In their case, the deceased was discovered with a hair dryer by her feet. Investigations concerning homicide were negative so a post-mortem examination was not carried out. Four years later, when murder was suspected, her body was exhumed and fractures to her hyoid bone and thyroid cartilage were found on radiography. She had apparently been manually strangled and then placed in the bath together with the hair dryer (presumably to deceive the investigators into thinking that they were dealing with an accidental or suicidal mode of death).

Road traffic accident scenes

The highway may be the site of discovery of a person thought to have been involved in a road traffic accident but where the death may be of a suspicious nature. In such cases a scene examination may reveal that:

1. The victim was intentionally fatally injured by a vehicle.
2. The victim had been struck by a car driven by someone who has committed an offence such as being over the legal limit for alcohol or under the influence of drugs.
3. The driver of the car had not stopped (hit and run driver) for whatever reason.
4. The victim had not been struck by a car but had been fatally wounded by some other means.

Boglioli et al. (1988) described an unusual vehicular suicide involving the driver leaning out through the side window of the moving vehicle so as to hit a highway sign stanchion. His upper torso was discovered under a highway sign next to tyre tread marks leading from the highway and continuing beyond the sign. The victim's lower torso and car were also found along the same path 31 m (101 ft) and 41 m (133 ft) beyond the sign, respectively. The deceased was initially thought to be a disposed homicide victim who had been dismembered by his assailants. Accident reconstruction, however, revealed that he had been transected by the sign stanchion as described above.

It should be appreciated that the motor vehicle is an ideal instrument of self-destruction for those intent on killing themselves. In examining the scene and vehicle, the following factors have been identified as significant in such cases: a vehicle collision with the middle of a fixed roadside object; an accelerator pedal mark on a shoe; the absence of skid marks; a witnessed acceleration into oncoming traffic. All the above should obviously be considered together with other relevant features such as: the presence of alcohol and/or drugs in significant quantities; appropriate psychiatric history; previous suicide attempts; suicide note or informing someone of suicide plans (Tillmann and Hobbs, 1949; Conger et al., 1957; Crancer and Quiring, 1969; Hollander, 1983; Hardwicke et al., 1985).

Drug related deaths

Scenes involving drug-related deaths, which may be treated as suspicious, fall into three broad categories involving:

1. Drugs of abuse.
2. Prescribed drugs and other medicines, usually related to overdose or adverse reaction.
3. Poisoning with other substances.

The most commonly encountered situations involve the first two categories.

In the case of an intravenous drug addict who is found dead, for example, the scene may not always appear to be straightforward. All the paraphenalia of drug abuse may have been cleared away by the deceased's associates and death made to appear 'natural'. On the other hand, if the person dies on their own, the situation is usually less complicated. A syringe may even be found still in the arm if death has been rapid. It is important to rule out any other cause of death, such as trauma resulting from an assault. The possibility of someone else injecting the drug into the deceased should also be borne in mind.

Occasionally, unusual presentations of drug suicides are encountered as in the two cases described by Hayman (1986), one of which is cited earlier in this chapter. In both cases, there were head injuries, which raised the possibility of homicide. It was postulated by the author that barbiturate poisoning may induce a phase of excitation, with headache, prior to the induction of coma.

References

Aguilar J. (1980) Forensic science investigation of a balloon accident. *J. For. Sci.* **25**, 522–527.

Boglioli L.R., Taff M.L., Green A.S., Lukash L.I. and Lane R. (1988) A bizarre case of vehicular suicide. *Am. J. For. Med. Pathol.* **9**, 169–178.

Conger J.J., Gaskill H.S., Gladd D.D., Rainey R.V., Sawrey W.L. and Turrell E.S. (1957) Personal and interpersonal factors in motor vehicle accidents. *Am. J. Psychiatry* **113**, 1069–1074.

Crancer A. Jr and Quiring D.L. (1969) The mentally ill as motor vehicle operators. *Am. J. Psychiatry* **126**, 807–813.

Devos C., Timperman J. and Piette M. (1985) Deaths in the bath. *Med. Sci. Law* **25**, 189–200.

Goonetilleke U.K.D.A. (1980) Injuries caused by falls from heights. *Med. Sci. Law* **20**, 262–275.

Hardwicke M.B. Taff M.L. and Spitz W.U. (1985) A case of suicidal hanging in an automobile. *Am. J. For. Med. Pathol.* **6**, 362–364.

Hayman J.A. (1986) Head injury associated with barbiturate suicide. *Am. J. For. Med. Pathol.* **7**, 78–80.

Hollander N. (1983) Motor vehicle suicides. In *Proceedings of the 16th Annual Meeting, American Association of Suicidology*, Dallas, Texas, p.123.

Lasczkowski G., Riepert T. and Rittner C. (1992) Zur Problematik des Auffindeortes Badewanne. Klarung eines Todesfalles nach vier Jahren unter Einsatz postmortaller Rontgendiagnostik. *Archiv Kriminol.* **189**, 25–32.

Leestma J.E., Teas S.S., Hughes J.R. and Kalelkar M.B. (1985) Sudden epilepsy deaths and the forensic pathologist. *Am. J. For. Med. Pathol.* **6**, 215–218.

McConnell T.S., Zumwalt R.E., Wah E.J., Haikal N.A. and McFeeley P.J. (1992) Rare electrocution due to power line contact in a hot air balloon: Comparison with fatalities from blunt trauma. *J. Foren. Sci.* **37**, 1393–1400.

Rabl W., Ambach E. and Tributsch W. (1990) Ungewohnliche Auffindungssituation eines Leichnams. Obduktions- und Ermittlungsergebnisse. *Archiv Kriminol.* **185**, 93–98.

Riddick L., Mussell G. and Cumberland G.D. (1989) The mirror's use in suicide. *Am. J. For. Med. Pathol.* **10**, 14–16.

Schmidt P., Haarhoff K. and Hoffmann E. (1991) Sekundar kombinierter Suizid unter den Augen der Ehefrau. *Archiv Kriminol.* **188**, 65–71.

Schwender L.A. and Troncoso J.C. (1986) Evaluation of sudden death in epilepsy. *Am. J. For. Med. Pathol.* **7**, 283–287.

Start R.D., Milroy C.M. and Green M.A. (1992) Suicide by self-stabbing. *For. Sci. Int.* **56**, 89–94.

Tillmann W.A. and Hobbs G.E. (1949) The accident-prone automobile driver: a study of the psychiatric and social background. *Am. J. Psychiatry* **106**, 321–331.

Vanezis P. and West I.E. (1983) Tentative injuries in self stabbing. *For. Sci. Int.* **21**, 65–70.

Wright R.K. (1983) Death or injury caused by electrocution. *Clin. Lab. Med.* **3**, 343–353.

Appendices

Appendices 1, 2 and 3 are from Lewington F. (1990) *Scenes of Crime – Information for Police Officers. Biology Notes.* Metropolitan Police Forensic Science Laboratory (copyright, Commissioner Metropolitan Police).

Handling, packaging and storage of blood-stained items

Type of sample	At the scene	Preferred packaging	General guidelines
1. Wet blood			**Wet blood**
• Large quantity	Remove with plastic pipette.	Bottle.	Allow to dry, in place, at room temperature (if feasible). Do not dry at police station. Otherwise package appropriately and submit to the laboratory at once. Delay in submission – refrigerate (do not freeze).
• Small quantity	Remove on tip(s) of dry cotton wool swabs.	Standard swab tube.	
2. Clotted blood	Scoop with spoon or spatula into tube/bottle		
3. Portable items/ clothing			
• Wet blood	Remove item.	Open polythene bag, transport to laboratory at once.	
			Dry blood
• Dry blood	Remove item.	Paper or polythene bag.	Store at room temperature.
4. Broken glass	Remove piece(s) of glass.	Cardboard box.	
5. Blood on wood, paint, plaster, paper, etc.	Remove stained area or whole item if appropriate (or scrape or swab as (10)).	Bottle, perspex box or tamper-proof bag.	**Container** Appropriate size for item. Sharp edges to be *safely* packaged.
6. Blood on soil	Transfer layer of soil intact to plastic tray.	On tray in paper bag. Submit at once.	Label appropriately and adequately.
7. Blood-stained vegetation	Remove blood-stained part, as (3).	Polythene or paper bag.	
8. Blood-stained carpet	As (3) or cut out stained fibres (+ unstained ones as control).	Polythene bag or bottle or perspex box.	**Controls** Control samples from an unstained area are required if an item is swabbed,
9. Small pieces flesh/bone/hair	Remove with forceps.	Bottle or screw-cap jar. Refrigerate.	scraped or only part of it is submitted. Controls should be packaged separately from
10. Dry blood on fixed surfaces			the blood stains.
• Large crusty stains	Scrape with scalpel.	Bottle or perspex box. Standard swab tube.	**Tamper-proof bags** Specially designed polythene
• Others	Remove on tip of moistened cotton wool swab.		bags for forensic exhibits. Use appropriate size of bag.
11. Knives	Pack immediately if blood is dry.	Cardboard box, secure knife safely to base.	

Handling, packaging and storage of semen-stained items

Type of sample	At the scene	Preferred packaging	Comments
1. Wet staining			
• Portable item	Remove item.	Paper bag.	Allow to dry in place
• Fixed surface	Cut out stained area (+ control unstained area) or remove on cotton wool swab (+ control swab).	Polythene bag or bottle. Standard swab tube. *Freeze.*	if possible. Package controls separately from stains.
2. Dry staining			
• Portable item	Remove item.	Paper bag.	Store at room
• Fixed surface	Cut out stained area (+ control unstained area) or scrape with a new scalpel into container.	Polythene bag or bottle. Bottle/perspex box.	temperature. Package controls separately.
• Vegetation stained with semen	Remove stained portion.	Paper bag.	Dry and store at room temperature or refrigerate.
• Soil stained with semen	Remove layer of soil onto tray.	On tray in paper bag.	Submit at once. Refrigerate meantime.

Handling, packaging and storage of entomological evidence

Life-cycle stage	Container	Food	Store
Eggs	Glass* universal bottle.	Small piece of body liver or muscle.	Room temperature or refrigerator. *Do not freeze.*
Larvae	Glass* universal bottle or capped glass* specimen jar.	Not too much food should be given nor too many larvae confined or larvae will drown in excessive moisture.	
Puparia	Glass* universal bottle.	None.	
Flies	Glass universal bottle.	None.	

*The seal should be removed and small holes punched in the cap for ventilation.

Scene of crime officers' (SOCO) standard equipment

2   SOCO aluminium cases
1   ESLA (electrostatic lifting apparatus) case (equipped)
2   Pairs green overalls
1   Waterproof jacket
1   Pair waterproof trousers
1   Pair steel capped boots
1   Helmet
1   Pair heavy duty vinyl gloves
1   Saw
1   Dustpan
1   Brush
1   Stanley knife
1   Measuring tape
1   Magnifying glass
1   Forensic footprint roller
1   Pair safety glasses
1   Polaroid camera
1   Lamp
1   Toolkit (tweezers, scalpel, etc.)
1   Geographia (street map)

All other scene and post-mortem supplies as per officers' own preference.

Index